W9-BPJ-309

FITBALL® WORKOUT

FITBALL® WORKOUT

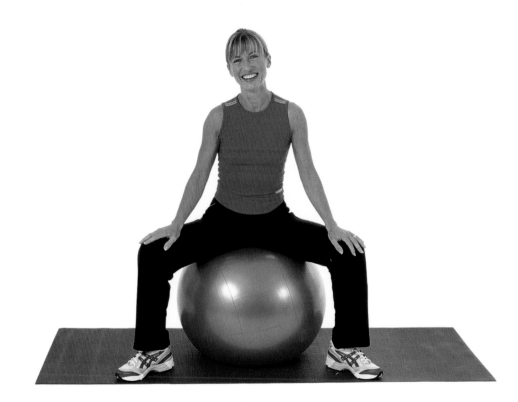

Jan Endacott

Select Editions

Jan Endacott trained for 12 years at the acclaimed Bush Davies Ballet School and subsequently travelled the world enjoying a successful career as a professional dancer and dance teacher. She then qualified as a personal fitness trainer and sports psychologist, creating her own unique exercise programme incorporating dance, yoga and Pilates techniques. Her enthusiasm for stability ball training has resulted in the development of the Fitball® Workout.

Fitball® (Europe) is a registered trademark belonging to
Ledraplastic Spa/Italy www.gymnic.com
Fitball® (USA) is a registered trademark belonging to
Ball Dynamics Int. Inc./Longmont CO www.balldynamics.com

Text copyright © Jan Endacott 2004
Book design copyright © Octopus Publishing Group Ltd 2004

This edition published in 2006 for
Select Publications
3918 Kitchener St
Burnaby BC Canada
V5C 3M2
www.selectpublications.ca

Tel: 604-415-2444
Fax: 604-415-3444

The right of Jan Endacott to be identified as the author of this work has been asserted by her in accordance with the Copyright, Designs and Patents Act, 1988.

All rights reserved. No part of this work may be reproduced or utilized in any form or by any means, electronic or mechanical, including photocopying, recording or by any information storage and retrieval system, without the prior written permission of the publisher.

ISBN 1-894905-71-7

A CIP catalogue record for this book is available from the British Library

Printed and bound in China

10 9 8 7 6 5 4 3 2 1

Note
Whilst the advice and information in this book is believed to be accurate, neither the author nor the publisher will be responsible for any injury, losses, damages, actions, proceedings, claims, demands, expenses and costs (including legal costs or expenses) incurred or in any way arising out of following the exercises in this book.

contents

introduction

The FitBall® is a large air-filled ball used for exercising at home. It's fun to use, versatile, amazingly effective and facilitates a workout that is so enjoyable that you could almost forget you are exercising! Even those people who are normally reluctant to exercise will become hooked on this comfortable way of achieving great results.

Benefits of using the ball

- The ball can be used in an extraordinary range of exercises that are suitable for all levels of fitness, from the unfit and overweight through to active sportsmen and sportswomen.

- Working with the ball allows you to concentrate on every muscle group, with the bonus that your postural muscles are constantly challenged. You can therefore target specific areas for firming and shaping, enabling you to achieve fantastic toning results for a leaner, more youthful body.

- Using the ball will improve your posture and strengthen your abdominal and back muscles. This enhances your overall core strength by continually training the deep stabilizing muscles that support your back.

- Greater flexibility is a major benefit. When particular muscles are stretched during an exercise, other muscles have to work to anchor and balance you on the ball. You can also achieve exercise positions unique to the ball that give a natural stretch to the spine and allow it to relax.

- The fitness training benefits of using the ball were originally recognized when it was used for treating patients with neuromuscular problems. It is widely acknowledged as a unique and valuable tool for developing strength, increasing flexibility, improving balance and enhancing co-ordination.

A variety of exercises

The range of exercises you will find in this book demonstrates the tremendous variety of ways in which the ball can be used. You can train lying or sitting on the ball, lying on the floor, standing, and even leaning on the ball against a wall.

Exercise intensity can be increased or decreased simply by adjusting the exercise position slightly. Because most start positions require your body to be balanced and stabilized on the ball, every exercise calls into play extra muscles that are not often challenged in floor or gym-machine-based exercises. Every routine is therefore extraordinarily effective and time-efficient, allowing you to achieve maximum results.

The cushioning support provided by the ball enables you to perform exercise variations that you may not have been able to attempt before, due to discomfort or underlying weakness. Working with the ball challenges muscles that normal daily activities just do not stimulate.

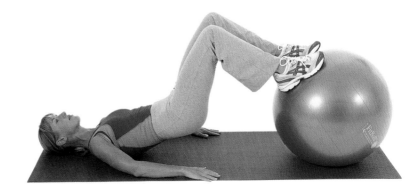

Achieving great results

As a result of exercising with the ball regularly, your body will be stronger and more flexible. This improved mobility and reduced muscular stiffness will help to reduce the risk of injury. As you age, it is essential to maintain flexibility and regular stretching, done using the ball, will help to improve your body's range of movement – a vital part in helping to prevent problems developing with your back, hips and knees. Greater flexibility and mobility also mean less stress will be placed on your joints.

It won't take long, once you're exercising regularly with your ball, before you notice that you stand tall and straight, helping you to feel younger, be stronger and appear visibly slimmer. Furthermore, you will enjoy the increased levels of vitality that are a result of feeling fit, healthy, poised and confident.

Whatever your age or current level of fitness, the workouts in this book will provide you with a choice of enjoyable non-impact exercises that will have you literally floating on air!

7

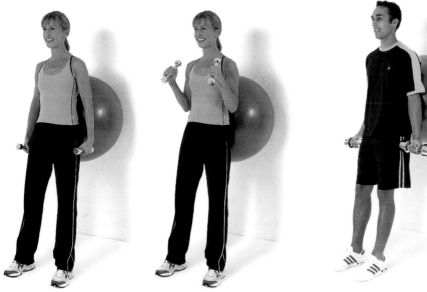
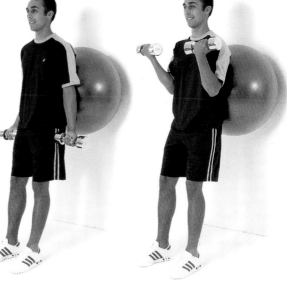

getting started

In your enthusiasm you may be tempted to dash into the nearest sports shop, grab a Fitball®, hurry home and start working out. Before you do, there are a few vital points you must consider. What size ball should you buy? How much should the ball be inflated? How do you exercise safely? The following advice will help you to achieve the very best results, in the safest possible way.

Choosing the correct ball size

When seated on the ball, your knees should be level with or slightly below your hips, with your knees bent at 90 degrees. Your feet should be flat on the floor. The following general guidelines will help you to determine the correct ball size for you. But, your height is not the only determining factor when selecting the correct ball size: your weight is also relevant.

- For overweight, unfit or more mature people, a larger ball that is used slightly under-inflated is usually preferable.
- It is also best to learn and practise new or more difficult exercises with the ball slightly under-inflated.
- A smaller, firmly inflated ball is more challenging to balance on than a larger, softer ball.

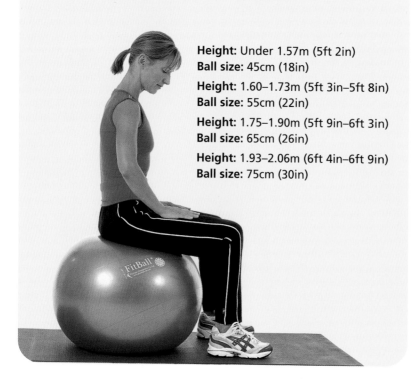

Height: Under 1.57m (5ft 2in)
Ball size: 45cm (18in)

Height: 1.60–1.73m (5ft 3in–5ft 8in)
Ball size: 55cm (22in)

Height: 1.75–1.90m (5ft 9in–6ft 3in)
Ball size: 65cm (26in)

Height: 1.93–2.06m (6ft 4in–6ft 9in)
Ball size: 75cm (30in)

Inflating the ball

You will need to use a hand or foot pump in conjunction with an appropriate adaptor to inflate the ball. Many stores that sell balls also keep special pumps in stock.

1 Leave the ball to reach room temperature before inflating.
2 Do not inflate past the ball's recommended maximum diameter. To check, simply measure the height of the ball from the floor. For example, a 65cm (26in) ball should not exceed a height of 65cm (26in). In some cases, under-inflating is acceptable (see box left).
3 Check the ball approximately once a month to ensure that the correct air-fill is maintained.

Exercise environment

- Make sure you have a clear floor space, with a clean and non-slip surface. The ideal exercising surface is a purpose-made exercise or yoga mat, available from most good sports stores.
- Wear suitable and comfortable exercise clothing (natural fibres are ideal), avoiding anything that restricts your freedom of movement.
- Store the ball at normal room temperature. DO NOT store the ball near any kind of heat source as this may melt the plastic.

Safety precautions

Before embarking on any new exercise programme, be honest with yourself. There is no benefit in aggravating an existing injury or medical condition, so study the advice below to enable you to proceed safely. You will then get the best from your exercising without any risk to your health.

Before you start

Always consult your doctor before starting this, or any, exercise programme, especially if any of the following apply:

- Your chest hurts when you are physically active.
- You have a heart condition.
- You have felt any chest pain recently when you are not doing physical activity.
- You suffer from loss of balance or dizzy spells or are prone to fainting.
- You suffer from high blood pressure.
- You have problems with your muscles, bones or joints that worsen when you are active.
- You are pregnant.

If you are not aware of any of the above, or any other reason you should not exercise, you can get started. However, it is essential to begin slowly and gradually so that your body can adapt to the demands placed upon it. Don't overdo it!

Exercising safely

- Always begin with a warm-up lasting about 5 minutes. Finish your workout with a minimum of 5 minutes of cool-down stretches.
- Avoid heavy weights if you suffer from raised blood pressure or any medical condition that may be aggravated by lifting.
- Remember to breathe: it is very common for people new to exercising to hold their breath.
- Pain means your body does not like something you are doing – so STOP! Do not work through pain: it is there to prevent you from causing yourself serious damage.
- It is unwise to exercise when you are ill. Your body is under attack and all your systems are fighting back, so you need all your reserves to help your body repair itself.
- Avoid exercise if you have drunk alcohol or are using any medication that may impair alertness.

Drinking and eating

Before and after exercising, make sure you have drunk enough fluid. If you feel thirsty, you are already dehydrated. Water is the body's temperature regulator and plays a vital role: drink at least 8 glasses a day, and even more when exercising, taking small sips at frequent intervals. Make sure you drink plenty after exercising to rehydrate your body. It's a good idea not to eat within 2 hours before exercising.

Don't forget to breathe

All ball exercises require you to pull your navel towards your spine. This is important because it stops the lower part of your stomach from rounding and popping up as you breathe in. Breathing correctly involves expanding your ribcage. Try it now! Breathe in through your nose and press your stomach flat whilst allowing your ribs to expand outwards. You should feel a stretch across your middle back. Now breathe out through your mouth making an audible blowing sound and flatten your stomach even more to help expel the air. Correct deep breathing takes practise – persevere! Deep breathing is good for detoxing because inhaling oxygen is energising, and breathing out fully gets rid of the stale air and toxins. Many of the exercises tell you when you should inhale and exhale. When there are no specific breathing instructions breathe using the above technique, keeping your abdominals pulled in throughout the exercise movements. Deep breathing is also a wonderful technique to use when relaxing and meditating.

training guidelines

The exercises in this book are designed to strengthen and tone all the muscles of your body with a balanced workout. One of the main aims of strength training is to increase lean muscle tissue: the more you have, the more effectively your body burns fat. This is because lean muscle tissue is active and 'eats up' calories, which are used to fuel the body's activities.

Take care

- **If you are pregnant, consult your doctor before embarking on any of the workout plans.**
- **Always leave a 48-hour rest period between workouts, because your muscles need some time in which to recover and repair themselves.**
- **Pay attention to how your body feels – it will tell you when it is tired.**
- **Remember: if something hurts – STOP!**

Lean muscle also helps you to burn up calories and fat long after you have finished exercising, because your metabolism remains higher for longer. This makes it the ideal mechanism for helping you to lose weight, feel more youthful and achieve a strong and toned body.

Using this book

The book begins with a series of warm-ups. You should perform these routines at the start of each exercise session to prepare your body and mind for the work ahead. The exercises are then arranged through the next three chapters according to the part of the body they are designed to help. Finally, the cool-down stretches will help to improve your flexibility, enhance relaxation and increase your vitality.

Choosing a workout plan

Various suggested workout plans are outlined on pages 120–125. Choose a plan to suit your needs and the time you have available. Ideally, you should aim to exercise 3 times a week, although you can break it down into 4 shorter sessions.

There are general full-body workouts for women and men, mature people or those who are less physically fit, and a back-care plan. The workouts are carefully balanced to achieve great results.

Reps and sets

A **repetition (rep)** is one complete cycle of an exercise: from the start position, through the whole sequence of movements, and back to the start position. The number of reps you should complete is specified for each exercise.

A **set** is the total number of reps you should complete continuously without a rest. For the majority of exercises, 1–3 sets are specified.

So, for example, if '5 reps/1 set' is specified, this means you should repeat the exercise sequence continuously 5 times before taking a break and then moving on to your next exercise. If your exercise should be done for '12 reps/2 sets', this means you should repeat the exercise sequence continuously 12 times before resting for 20–30 seconds, then perform the sequence continuously another 12 times.

Depending on your level of fitness when you start, decide how many sets you can manage. At the beginning this will generally be 1 or 2 sets, moving on to 3 sets when you find 2 sets easy. Always remember to rest between sets.

The megachallenge

Some of the exercises have a 'megachallenge' variation. This provides you with a much more demanding exercise to try when the standard version no longer seems enough for you. Do not attempt any megachallenge until you are performing the standard version with ease. Unless otherwise stated, the number of reps and sets for the megachallenge is the same as for the standard exercise.

Selecting dumb-bells

Ideally, you should buy 3 sets of dumb-bells: light, medium and heavy. The medium dumb-bell weight for you will be one you can lift continuously 12 times when performing a Biceps Curl (see page 50). You should also buy a pair of

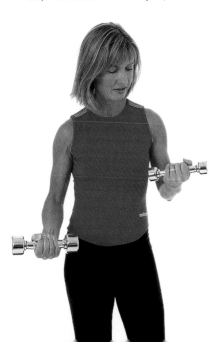

dumb-bells 1kg (2¼lb) lighter and a pair 1kg (2¼lb) heavier.

These 3 weights will accommodate all the dumb-bell exercises in this book and ensure you work all your muscles at the correct level. The appropriate weight for each exercise will be the one you can lift continuously for the required number of reps, with the last 2 reps being an effort to complete. As you progress and become stronger, you will probably need to invest in some heavier dumb-bells.

When to exercise

Choose a time to exercise and then stick to it! Exercising first thing in the morning is often best, as it gets you off to a flying start for the day. Gain the extra time you need by setting your alarm clock for a couple of minutes earlier every day, thereby easing yourself into the earlier start gradually. This way, it will be less of a shock to your system. Start a fitness diary (see page 13) and note down the time you start each morning to help you stay on track.

Aerobic exercise

For complete fitness, you must do some form of daily aerobic exercise in addition to your ball workout to keep

> **TRAINER'S TIPS**
> ❶ Build your strength gradually.
> ❷ Always put in 100 per cent effort.
> ❸ Concentrate completely on what you are doing – not on what you are going to do after your workout!

your heart strong and your lungs healthy. Your heart is like any other muscle: if it's not given a workout it will become lazy.

The easiest aerobic exercise is walking. Aim for at least 20 minutes daily, building up to 30 minutes. Walk briskly with a purpose, swinging your arms with a controlled, pumping action. Be realistic, though: if you can only manage 3 minutes, that's fine. Just build up gradually – it's better than no minutes at all. What's more, you can walk at any time of day.

Other aerobic non-impact activities you may want to try are swimming and cycling, both of which are easy on your joints. For the more energetic person, skipping with a rope is extremely effective.

Losing weight

Here is a simple fact: to lose weight, you have to create what's known as a calorie deficit. If you eat more calories than your body requires for activity, they will be stored as fat.

Diet

Balance your exercise with a healthy diet. Eat at regular times and never skip meals. Eat less in the evening, because what you don't use as fuel for activity will be stored as fat. Eat fresh organic, unrefined and unprocessed foods whenever possible. This will help you to avoid hidden salts, bad fats and chemically treated foods. Keep to a modest intake of caffeine and alcohol.

setting goals

For any health and exercise programme to be successful, you must set yourself clearly defined goals. For example, your ultimate aim might be to lose your 'spare tyre' and achieve a firm, flat stomach. Whatever you decide, you must be specific. You must not only identify what you really want but also how you are going to get there. Write your goals down in your fitness diary – make them real. Writing is a positive action and makes you really think about what you are doing.

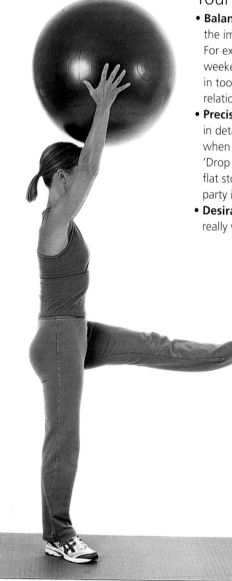

Your goals must be:

- **Balanced** They must cater for all the important aspects of your life. For example, devoting your whole weekend to exercising may not fit in too well with your personal relationship. Be realistic!
- **Precise** Describe and write down in detail what you really want, and when you want it by. For example: 'Drop 2 dress sizes and achieve a flat stomach in time for the office party in 4 months' time'.
- **Desirable** They must be what you really want.
- **Challenging** Your goals should push you to improve yourself.
- **Time-framed** It's essential to have an 'achieve-by' date, otherwise you will end up drifting along aimlessly.

All this will compel you to clarify and be realistic about your ultimate aims and desires of your workout plan.

Long- and short-term goals

Identify your long-term goals first. For example, you may want to be fit enough in 12 months' time to take part in a non-competitive marathon. Writing down this long-term goal will turn it into a concrete ambition, help you commit to it and define your aims clearly. Make your long-term goals specific and precise, and write down every detail as you imagine it. You will then have a clear picture of how fantastic it will be when you get there.

Now write down your short-term goals. Think of these as stepping-stones that form the path along the way to your long-term goals. It is easier if you break this down initially into monthly targets, then plan two or three achievements per week. This way, you can measure your success weekly. Tick off your targets as soon as you achieve them so that you can see your progress.

12

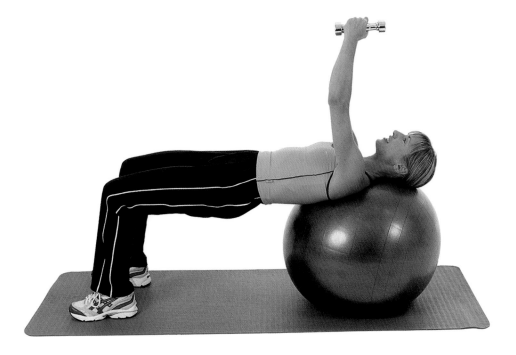

Keeping a fitness diary

The aim of writing in a diary every day is to help you chart your progress. After every workout, write down the ball exercises you have completed, then add any daily aerobic activity such as walking.

If your goal is weight loss, for the first week or two it is a good idea to keep a food diary to help you identify slip-ups and avoid energy slumps.

Visualization and music

Visualization is one of the most effective methods of using the power of your mind to affect physical performance and results.

- Keep imagining what it will be like when you have achieved your goals. Think about all the compliments you will receive and how good that will feel.
- Think of all the positive steps you are taking to achieve your goals.
- Use visualization with each exercise; for example, imagine the movement before you perform it. This will help you achieve a sound technique and better end results.

Using background music is another way of helping you to achieve your goals. Listening to music you enjoy as you exercise allows you to experience positive thoughts and feelings, which in turn will help you to feel more motivated and achieve better results.

All these techniques can work for you, and with perseverance you will master things you may previously have thought were impossible. Remember to stay focused and prepare to build the new you!

13

Review your goals

- **If you miss a goal, don't panic! Revise and redefine your goals as you move on.**
- **Be disciplined. Reviewing your goals on a regular basis helps to remind you exactly what it is you want to achieve and reinforces the idea of where you are heading.**

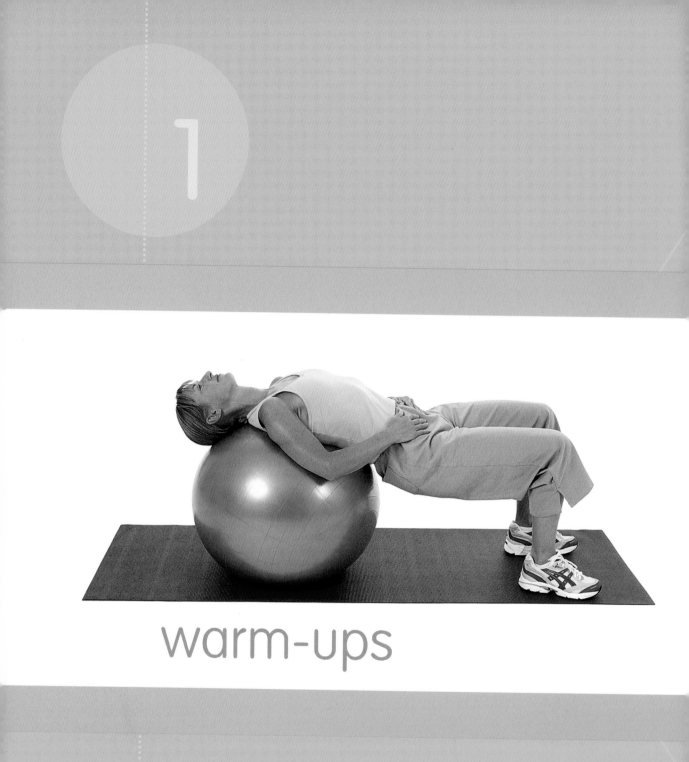

warm-ups

The purpose of warming up is to prepare your body for the exercising to come. During a warm-up, your body temperature and heart rate are raised, your muscles are warmed, oxygen consumption is increased and your joints are loosened. Most importantly, all these factors reduce the possibility of injury.

The warming-up part of your workout is also the perfect time for mental preparation. It's a good idea to leave behind the worries of the day and focus your thoughts on you and your workout. During your workout concentrate on the area of your body that you are exercising. To be effective and avoid the risk of injury, perform all the movements at a slow to moderate pace. Remain focused and in control, and maintain good posture and technique throughout.

If you do not want to do all your warm-up on the ball, try marching on the spot and swinging your arms for several minutes. Then perform a few of the warm-up exercises with the ball.

On pages 23–29 you will find some simple stretches. These are not essential for warming up, but many people prefer to do them because it helps them to feel more fully prepared, both physically and mentally. Apply these stretches to the main muscles you intend to exercise.

Generally, the fitter you are, the less warm-up time you need. However, never do less than 4–5 minutes. Begin with the postural awareness exercises on page 16 to familiarize yourself with positioning, then start at the top of your body and work through each area in turn.

Neutral Spine

reps	sets
1	1

A 'neutral' spine refers to the natural curves of the spine. By adopting this position you will avoid having to force the curves of your back into uncomfortable contortions. This is a good exercise for improving postural awareness.

➡ This is your neutral spine position. Try to avoid slouching your shoulders, tilting your pelvis or arching your back.

Body Balancer

reps	sets
1	1

The Body Balancer opens your upper body and chest area, creating increased awareness of your abdominal area.

> **TRAINER'S TIPS**
> ❶ **Caution!** If your neck feels tense or you find this position uncomfortable, place one hand behind your head for support.

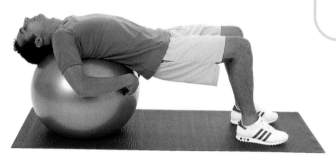

⬅ Sit on the ball and walk your feet out, breathing in as you do so, until your head is completely relaxed on the ball. Use your abdominal muscles to hold your stomach firm.

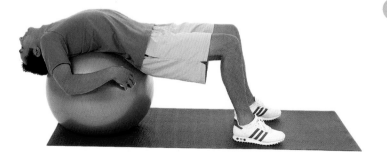

⬅ Use your buttocks and the backs of your legs to help keep your pelvis up. Walk your feet in slightly, allowing your head and back to extend backwards over the ball. Breathe out as you return to the start position, contracting your stomach muscles and pulling your navel in towards your spine. Drop your chin down slightly and come into an upright position, walking your feet back in.

Ab-Engager: Abs to Back

reps	sets
5–6	1

Mastering the three positions on this page will help you learn how to activate the postural muscles that support your back. This exercise engages the deep abdominal muscles, which run like a corset around your middle. Training them will flatten your stomach.

Place your hands like a fan across the lower part of your stomach. Breathe in, and as you breathe out pull your stomach away from your hands. Release.

Ab-Engager: Ribs to Hips

reps	sets
4–5	1

This exercise teaches you to activate the oblique muscles that control your rib cage and pelvis. Understanding how to draw your ribs and hips together is essential for effective abdominal work.

Breathe in to prepare, then breathe out as you slide your ribs down towards your hips. Breathe in as you return to a neutral spine position (see opposite).

17

Ab-Engager: Recumbent Ribs to Hips

reps	sets
4–5	1

This exercise is an effective preparation for the start position of Abs-olutely Fabulous (see page 68).

Practise the previous exercise lying back on the ball with your hips dropped. Imagine holding an orange under your chin to stop your head rolling back. Breathe in, then as you breathe out draw your ribs towards your hips. Release to the neutral spine position.

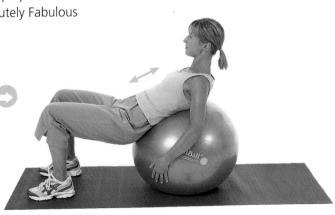

Shoulder Rolls

reps	sets
6–8	2

This movement mobilizes and prepares the shoulder muscles and, if done regularly, can increase mobility and enhance your postural awareness. In addition, Shoulder Rolls will encourage your chest to open because it relaxes your shoulder muscles. Tense shoulders cause a rounded upper back and bad posture.

Sit upright on the ball. Pull your navel in towards your spine to stabilize your back. Look straight ahead and relax your shoulders.

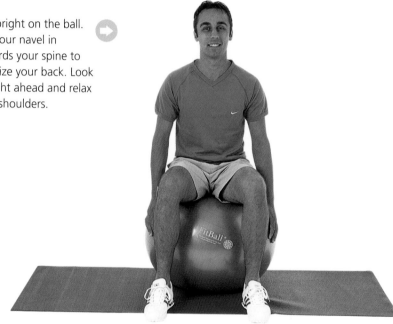

Slowly lift and roll your shoulders backwards, drop them down and then return to the start position. Perform one set. Now do the same shoulder lift, but this time roll your shoulders forwards, drop them down and then return once more to the start position. Perform one set.

TRAINER'S TIPS
1 Relax your hands as you circle your shoulders.
2 Pull your navel in towards your spine throughout.

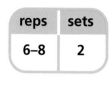

Ball Bounce

reps	sets
8–10	1–2

This warm-up exercise is huge fun and will bring a smile to your face! Practised in a controlled manner, it will help to increase general mobility in your spinal discs and will also improve your coordination skills.

Sit upright on the ball. Position your knees over your feet, and place your hands to the sides of the ball. Pull your navel in towards your spine and bounce on the ball.

Bouncing Jacks

reps	sets
8–10	1–2

A more demanding version of the Ball Bounce, this exercise will make the bounce more intense and really challenge your coordination. It will also increase your range of movement and work your shoulder muscles.

From the same start position as the Ball Bounce, lift your arms above your head and bounce, then lower your arms and bounce, to complete 1 rep.

TRAINER'S TIP
Pull your navel in towards your spine to keep a strong centre. Never let your centre collapse.

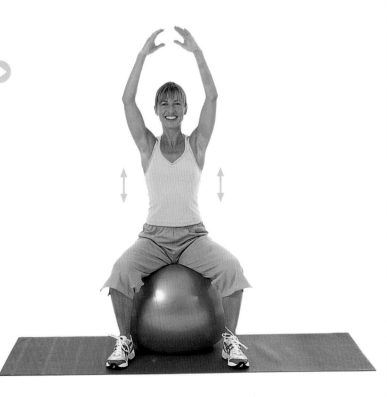

Twisters

reps	sets
6–8	1

This exercise will mobilize your upper body muscles and improve your posture, by forcing you to lift up and out of your hips. Using the muscles that twist and turn your body will prepare you for the core-strengthening exercises to come and will help you to hold yourself upright naturally.

Sit upright on the ball. Place your arms in front of you at shoulder height, bending your elbows and resting one hand on top of the other. Keep your body lifted and your hips still. Your hips must remain square to the front.

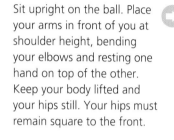

20

Turn slowly from your waist upwards and look over your right shoulder. Hold for a second, then return to the centre. Lift up tall and turn to look over your left shoulder. Your hips must face the front throughout.

TRAINER'S TIPS
❶ Think of your abdominal muscles wrapping around your middle like a corset, holding your stomach firm.
❷ Pull your navel in towards your spine throughout.

Rock'n'Roll

reps	sets
6–8	1

This pelvis-rocking exercise is good for improving general mobility in your lower back and pelvis. It is a relaxing movement to do and really prepares your lower spine for the strengthening exercises to come.

Sit upright on the ball with your spine in a neutral position (see page 16). Position your knees over your feet and place your hands on your hips. Now roll the ball forwards as you tilt your hips backwards.

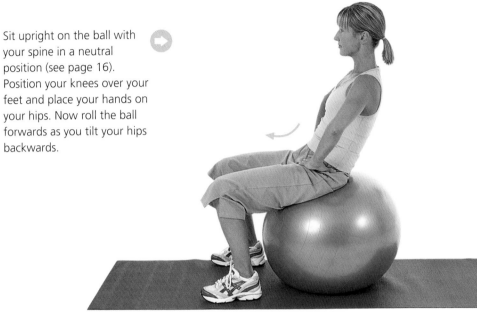

Now come back through the neutral spine position and roll the ball backwards as you tilt your hips forwards. Your back will naturally arch slightly. Return to the start position with a neutral spine.

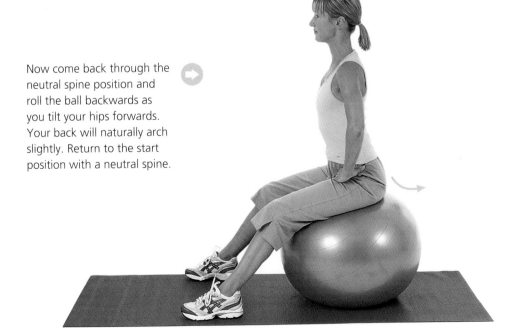

Revolver

reps	sets
8	1

This effective preparation movement improves flexibility in the spine and hip area. You can use this as a warm-up before exercise, or to mobilize and remove tension any time you feel stiff. It is particularly beneficial for people in desk-bound jobs or who spend hours in the driving seat.

Sit on the ball, with your knees over your feet and hands on your thighs. Make a circular movement with your hips, rotating them clockwise for 8 circles, then anticlockwise for another 8 circles. This completes 1 set.

TRAINER'S TIPS
1. Imagine drawing the circles in your head as your hips rotate.
2. Try not to exaggerate the circles, which compromises good technique.

Revolving '8'

reps	sets
8	1

This is a challenging pelvic-rotation exercise. It requires good concentration to focus on co-ordination: Revolving '8' is a 'wake-up' for the mind!

Sit upright on the ball as in the Revolver. Make a figure-of-eight shape with your hips, moving them in even circles; perform one circle in one direction and one circle in the opposite direction to complete a repetition. Pull your navel in towards your spine throughout.

Rainbow

reps	sets
4–5	1

This stretch increases flexibility in your torso. The gentle lengthening movement improves your awareness of the central girdle and postural muscles, and works your waist muscles. It also helps alleviate backache by gently lengthening your spine.

Sit upright, keeping your buttocks anchored on the ball and your knees over your feet. Pull your navel in towards your spine. Raise one arm over your head and rest the opposite hand on your thigh.

TRAINER'S TIPS
1 Pull your body up out of your hips. This provides a terrific waist workout.
2 Keep your head and neck in alignment with your spine; look straight ahead.

23

Lift and lengthen towards the ceiling, then reach across and over as far as is comfortable. Allow the hand resting on your thigh to shift naturally and rest your elbow. Pull up through your centre and return to the start position. Repeat up to 5 times on each side to complete 1 set.

Rear Leg Stretch

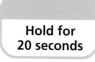

Hold for 20 seconds

This stretch is great preparation for the leg work to follow and also before your aerobic exercise. It stretches your calf muscle as well as the hamstrings (back of your thigh) and releases any muscle tension. Strong, flexible hamstrings can help alleviate lower-back stiffness and guard against injury.

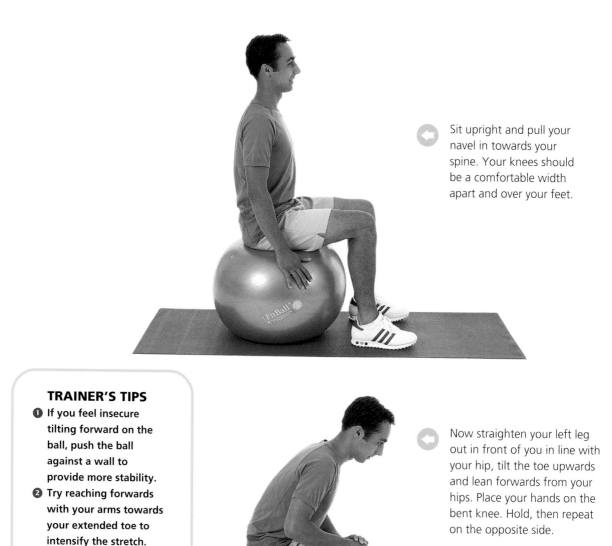

Sit upright and pull your navel in towards your spine. Your knees should be a comfortable width apart and over your feet.

TRAINER'S TIPS
1. If you feel insecure tilting forward on the ball, push the ball against a wall to provide more stability.
2. Try reaching forwards with your arms towards your extended toe to intensify the stretch.

Now straighten your left leg out in front of you in line with your hip, tilt the toe upwards and lean forwards from your hips. Place your hands on the bent knee. Hold, then repeat on the opposite side.

Leg Lengthener

Hold for 20 seconds

This is a good stretch for the quadriceps muscles at the front of your thighs and is good preparation for ball exercises or aerobic work. A lot of strength work focuses on these muscles and regular stretches help to lengthen the appearance of the muscle, keeping it long and lean.

Sit on the ball and slowly walk your feet out until your head, neck and shoulders rest on the ball. Place your hands on your hips while pulling your navel towards your spine. Your knees should be over your feet.

TRAINER'S TIPS
❶ Stay lifted up underneath your buttocks to avoid them sinking towards the floor.
❷ Pull your navel in towards your spine to stabilize your back throughout.

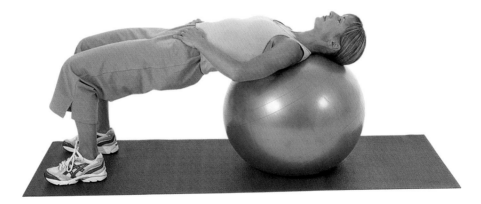

Slide the heel of your left leg back towards the ball, keeping the heel lifted from the floor. Hold, then repeat on the other side.

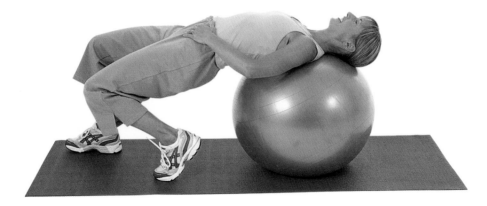

Hip Lunge

This excellent stretch loosens and prepares the muscles at the front of your hips. The hip-flexor muscles are often neglected in warm-ups, and yet they are of vital importance because they can shorten, contributing to lower-back discomfort. This stretch will improve the range of movement in your hip area. It is ideal for people who spend hours sitting at a desk or driving.

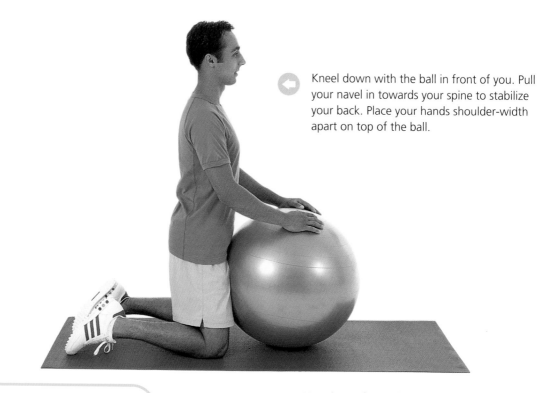

Kneel down with the ball in front of you. Pull your navel in towards your spine to stabilize your back. Place your hands shoulder-width apart on top of the ball.

TRAINER'S TIP
Avoid over-stretching. You must always feel comfortable when you stretch.

Now lunge forwards with your left knee bent around the ball, positioning the ball underneath your stomach. Bring your right leg backwards and straighten it out. Hold, then repeat on the other side.

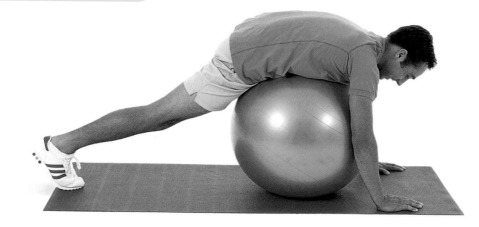

26

Upper-Back Stretch

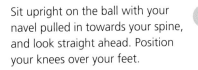

Hold for 10 seconds

This stretch relieves general stiffness and tension and increases general flexibility. It is good before exercise and particularly before upper-body work. This is an easy everyday stretch, useful for people who sit still for long hours or do lots of gardening (prolonged bending) or anyone who regularly carries heavy loads.

Sit upright on the ball with your navel pulled in towards your spine, and look straight ahead. Position your knees over your feet.

Straighten your arms in front of you and clasp your hands away from you, holding your upper body firm. Hold.

TRAINER'S TIPS

❶ You should feel this stretch right across your upper back and in the backs of your shoulders.

❷ Avoid hunching your shoulders: keep them relaxed as you breathe slowly and evenly while you hold the stretch.

Seated Chest Opener

Hold for 10 seconds

This chest stretch opens the whole area across the front of your upper body and is an essential movement to maintain strength and flexibility in this area. Your chest can easily store tension, which in turn produces stiff muscles and postural weakness. Regular stretching helps to prevent tension in your chest.

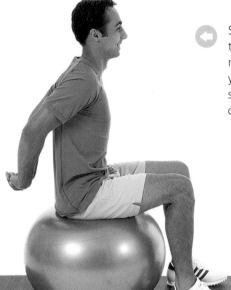

Sit upright on the ball with your navel pulled in firmly towards your spine, keeping your head, neck and shoulders relaxed. Clasp your hands behind your back and lengthen your spine. Raise your arms slightly without hunching your shoulders until you can feel a stretch developing across your chest area.

28

Kneeling Chest Opener

Hold for 10 seconds

Another good stretch for the chest, this position enables you to work each side of the chest separately, thereby providing an effective alternative stretch.

Kneel down beside the ball, placing your right hand on it and your left hand on the floor just in front of you. Roll the ball directly out to the side of your body. Gently press your shoulder downwards towards the floor. Hold, then repeat with the other arm.

TRAINER'S TIPS
1. Pull your navel in towards your spine to prevent your back dipping.
2. Keep your weight evenly distributed on both knees and avoid twisting off-centre.

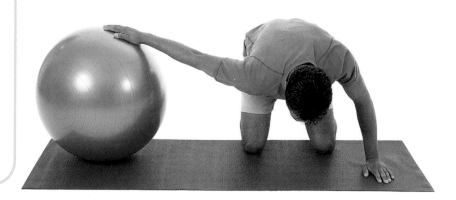
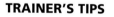

Look Away

**Hold for
10 seconds**

Effectively stretching your shoulder muscles, this exercise will also stretch your chest. It is common for tension to be stored in the shoulder area, particularly if you are working at a computer. The chest is also prone to storing tension, so flexible muscles in this region will help to prevent postural problems.

Sit on the ball and walk your feet out until the ball cushions your back. Your head, neck and shoulders should be supported and your hands should rest lightly on your stomach.

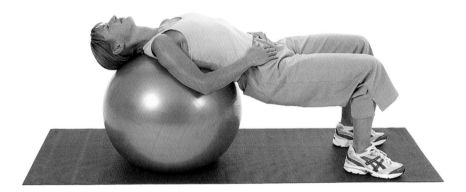

29

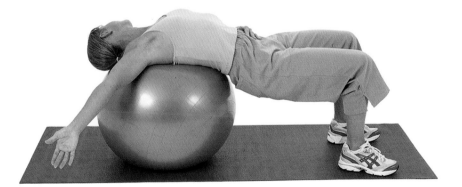

TRAINER'S TIPS
❶ Make sure your back is fully cushioned on the ball.
❷ Your head should rest on the ball but not overhang.

Extend your right arm over your head and turn your palm up and out, turning your head to look in the opposite direction. Hold, then repeat on the other side.

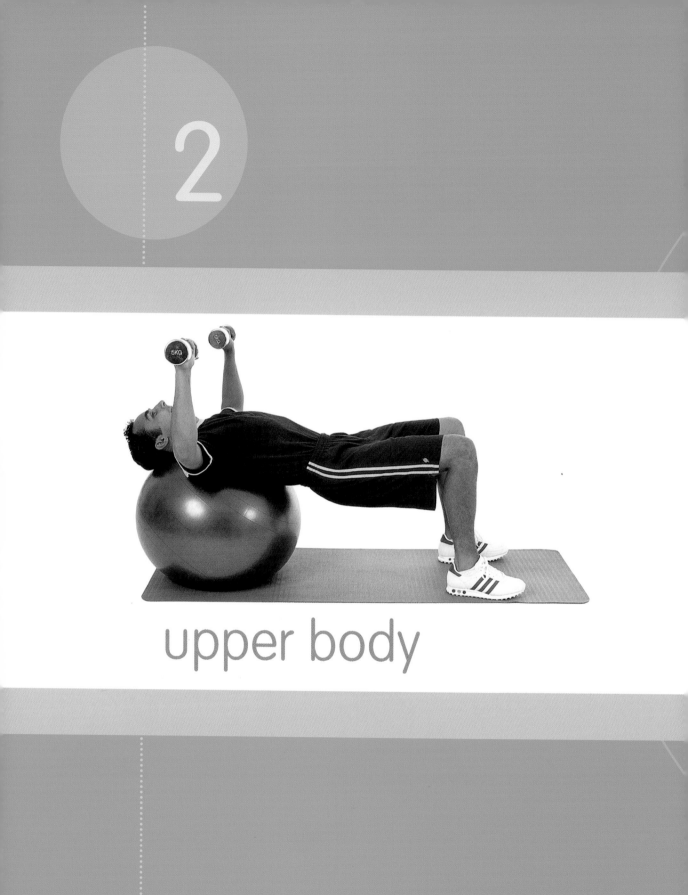

upper body

This chapter focuses on your body from the waist up. However, beware of exercising just one part of your upper body – you will not only create muscular imbalance, which can lead to injury, but may also finish up looking rather odd! A balanced approach is best: training your upper body involves exercising your upper back, chest, shoulders and arms.

For women, toned arms and shoulders are attractive, while firmer chest muscles improve bust shape. An attractive upper body draws focus away from your lower half if you are pear-shaped, helping to create a more balanced look.

A common problem area is the backs of the arms, which easily lose their shape and can become flabby. Rescue is at hand with regular exercises targeted at the triceps muscle. Be assured that you will not bulk up, as women do not have the testosterone necessary to achieve this.

Men will gain strength and increased muscle size from a balanced upper-body workout. They will need to use much heavier weights than women and will probably find the more intense levels and megachallenges useful as they progress. The result: a broader chest, a strong, well-defined upper back and muscular arms.

Looking and feeling good are benefits of regular exercise, but the main objective is to become fitter and stronger. Each of the exercises here has been chosen for its effectiveness, and there are some that are crucial to correct posture and eliminate rounded shoulders.

Wheelbarrow

reps	sets
4	1

This is an essential preparation exercise. Practising this movement provides a sound technique for the Ball Press-Up on page 38. The Wheelbarrow improves strength and power in your entire upper body, especially the shoulder muscles. You will also be challenging your lower abdominal muscles and mid-back area, which will enhance core stability.

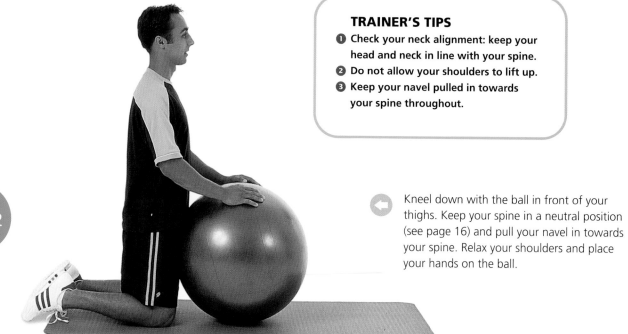

> **TRAINER'S TIPS**
> ❶ Check your neck alignment: keep your head and neck in line with your spine.
> ❷ Do not allow your shoulders to lift up.
> ❸ Keep your navel pulled in towards your spine throughout.

Kneel down with the ball in front of your thighs. Keep your spine in a neutral position (see page 16) and pull your navel in towards your spine. Relax your shoulders and place your hands on the ball.

Lean forward over the ball until your hands touch the floor and the ball supports your body weight. Feel how pushing into your hands supports your weight.

Push out over the ball, walking your hands out so that the ball is underneath your thighs. Keep your navel pulled in towards your spine to help keep your hips and lower back straight. Walk your hands back in towards the ball.

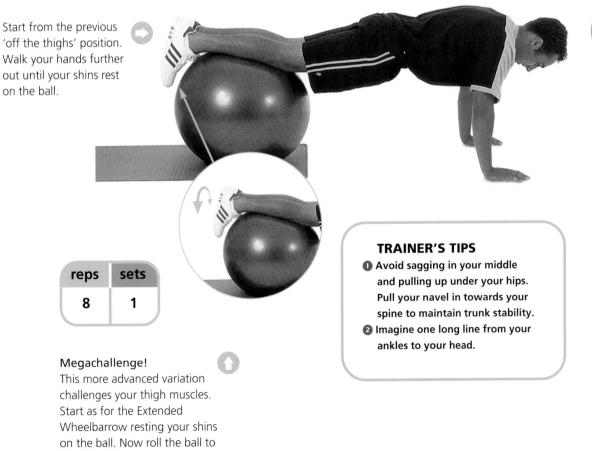

Extended Wheelbarrow

reps	sets
4	1

The Extended Wheelbarrow increases the body leverage. Attempt this version only when you feel you have mastered the basic Wheelbarrow position.

Start from the previous 'off the thighs' position. Walk your hands further out until your shins rest on the ball.

reps	sets
8	1

TRAINER'S TIPS
❶ Avoid sagging in your middle and pulling up under your hips. Pull your navel in towards your spine to maintain trunk stability.
❷ Imagine one long line from your ankles to your head.

Megachallenge!
This more advanced variation challenges your thigh muscles. Start as for the Extended Wheelbarrow resting your shins on the ball. Now roll the ball to one side (1 rep), then the other.

Walkaway

reps	sets
4	1

This sequence is good preparation for many exercises, particularly those that use dumb-bells and require good control. Practise the Walkaway before attempting any of the upper-body exercises that begin from this start position. Your buttock muscles work with your abdominals to improve the strength in your torso and pelvis. Practise slowly and make sure you hold the end position.

Begin in a seated position on the ball. Pull up tall from the top of your head. Pull your navel in towards your spine and keep your spine in a neutral position (see page 16). Your neck and shoulders should remain relaxed, with a feeling of breadth across your chest.

With your hands resting on your hips, slowly walk your feet away from the ball. Tuck in your chin as you walk your feet out and scoop your stomach to curve your spine.

TRAINER'S TIPS
1. Imagine the shape of an ice-cream scoop, and think of this when you are scooping your stomach inwards.
2. Keep your chin tucked in as you walk out.

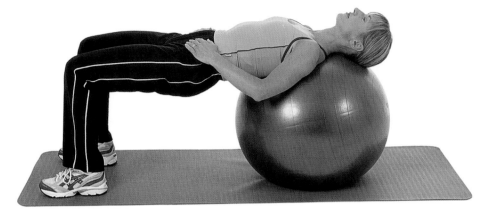

⬆ Continue to walk away from the ball until your shoulders come to rest on it. Your head and neck should feel comfortable on the ball. With your stomach pulled in and your spine in a neutral position, anchor and support your body by using your buttock muscles.

⬇ To return to the start position, simply reverse the movement and walk your feet towards the ball. The body curve begins by tucking from your chin, then pulling your navel in towards your spine to control your torso and maintain a taut stomach.

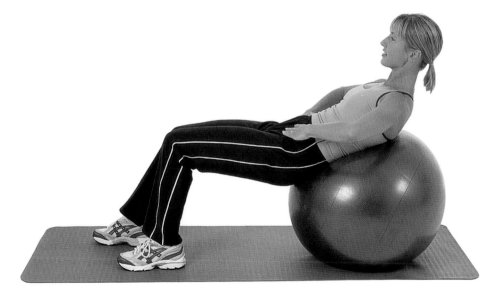

TRAINER'S TIPS
1 When your shoulders rest on the ball, avoid tucking in your chin or tilting it up.
2 Visualize keeping your neck lengthened.
3 Visualize your scooped-out stomach during the movement.
4 Push your back into the ball as you return to an upright position.

Drifter

reps	sets
8–10	1

This exercise focuses on your body alignment, using the main muscles in your torso to improve core strength and hip stability. The Drifter enhances concentration and is a good preparation movement to practise before the dumb-bell exercises. The movement of the ball enables you to practise transference of body weight.

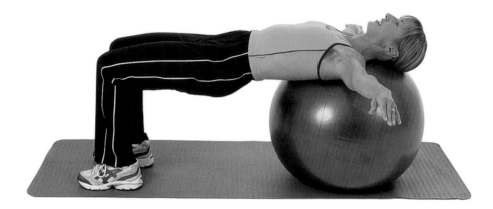

Start in the Walkaway position. Rest your shoulders on the ball, your neck and lower spine will be in a neutral position (see page 16). Extend your arms out sideways from your shoulders and maintain control of your torso by pulling your navel firmly towards your spine.

Shift your weight across the ball to the left. Maintain body and hip alignment and keep your feet still. The ball will roll underneath your shoulders and out to your right side, while your body weight will transfer to your left buttock. Move back to the centre to complete 1 rep. Repeat on the opposite side. Return to the sitting position as for the Walkaway.

TRAINER'S TIPS
1. Use your stomach and buttock muscles to anchor your torso.
2. Keep your legs still. Do not let your knees move in the opposite direction to your shoulders.

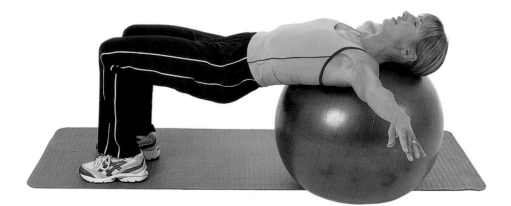

Chest Flyes

reps	sets
8–12	1–3

This exercise is a great way to improve the strength and shape of your chest and will help to firm the muscles that lift the bust. Chest Flyes use the ball as a bench to support your shoulders, neck and head. Make sure you can do the Walkaway (see pages 34–35) before tackling this exercise.

Select suitable weights (see page 11), then start in the Walkaway position. Holding a dumb-bell in each hand, extend your arms straight above your head. Keep your elbows slightly bent with your palms facing each other. Look straight up. Keep your knees over your feet and use your buttocks to steady you.

Breathe in as you carry your arms outwards until they are almost parallel with the floor. Breathe out as you bring your arms towards each other, feeling your chest muscles contracting as they do so.

TRAINER'S TIPS
1 Pull your navel in towards your spine to stabilize your back.
2 Keep a slight bend on your elbows to prevent them locking.

37

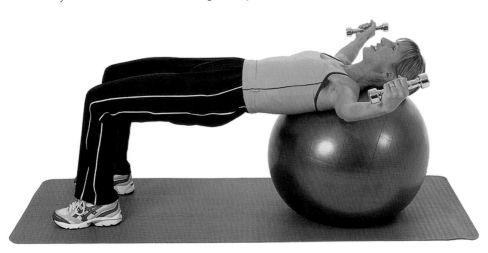

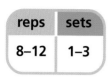

Ball Press-Up

reps	sets
8–12	1–3

This versatile exercise improves strength in the chest, shoulders and backs of the arms, with the bonuses of challenging your abdominal muscles and improving your balance skills.

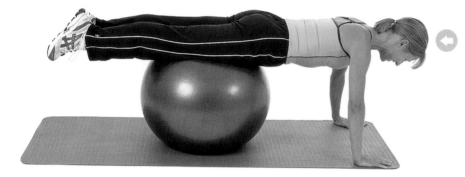

Begin with your stomach on the ball. Walk your hands forward until your thighs rest on it (practise the Wheelbarrow on pages 32-33). Place your hands under your shoulders with slightly bent elbows and fingers pointing forwards. Pull your navel in towards your spine to hold your back in alignment.

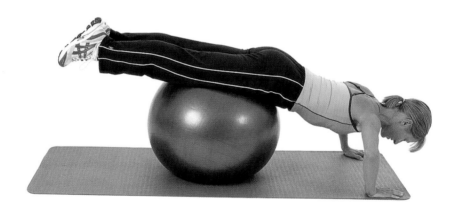

Breathing in, bend your elbows at 90 degrees as you lower your body. Keep your head in line with your back. Keep your stomach and thighs firm and your legs straight. Breathing out, push back up to the start position.

TRAINER'S TIPS
1. Avoid lifting your buttocks.
2. For increased emphasis on your chest area, place your hands slightly further apart.
3. Correct breathing helps your abdominals contract fully, ensuring good technique.

Wall Press-Up

reps	sets
8–12	1–3

This is a good starting point if you are unfit, overweight or recovering from a shoulder injury. Its intensity is controlled by the distance you place your feet from the ball. The further away, the more difficult the movement.

Hold the ball against the wall with your arms stretched out at shoulder level. If you feel discomfort in your lower spine, bend your arms more. Bend your elbows and lean towards the ball, then straighten your elbows to return to the start position.

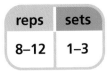

Off-Toes Press-Up

reps	sets
8–12	1–3

This works the same muscles, but with the main focus shifted towards the middle of your chest.

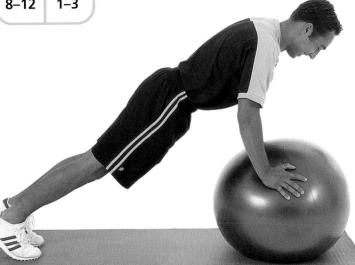

Start with your body straight and your toes on the floor. Hold the ball on either side, with your hands placed under your shoulders. Squeeze the ball to hold it steady.

Breathe in as you bend your elbows to lower down to the ball, holding your body in a straight line. Keep the movement slow and controlled. Breathe out as you push back up.

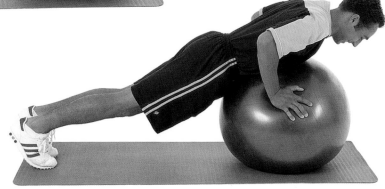

39

Chest Press

reps	sets
8–12	1–3

This is an effective exercise that will tone and shape the chest and backs of the arms. Use it as an alternative to press-ups. Ensure you are familiar with the Walkaway exercise (see pages 34–35) before you try this, as you are using the ball as a bench.

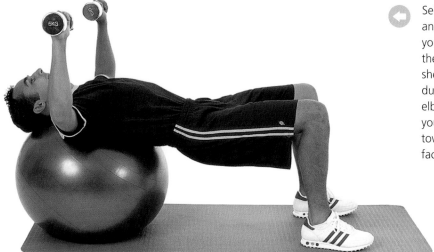

Select suitable weights (see page 11) and rest them on your thighs. Walk your feet out from the ball until only the base of your head, neck and shoulders are on the ball. With a dumb-bell in each hand, bend your elbows to 90 degrees – in line with your chest. Your knuckles now point towards the ceiling and your palms face forwards. This is the start position.

40

TRAINER'S TIPS
❶ Pull your navel towards your spine to stabilize your back.
❷ Use your buttocks to raise your hips and maintain good alignment
❸ Avoid flexing your wrists.

Push the dumb-bells upwards using slow, controlled movements, until your arms are nearly straight; do not lock your elbows. Hold for a second, then return to the start position. Breathe out as you press the dumb-bells upwards, breathe in as you return to the start position.

Arm Circles

reps	sets
16	2

This is a great exercise for sculpting the whole upper-arm area while strengthening the upper back. It will also provide a good stretch for forearm and wrist muscles and will strengthen the muscles around your shoulder joints without placing stress on the joints themselves. Tensing your buttock muscles will help you to maintain stability on the ball.

Sit upright and pull your navel in towards your spine. Hold your arms out at shoulder height. Flex and extend your wrists, pushing into the heels of your hands. Circle your arms forwards 8 times and then backwards 8 times to complete 1 set. Use small and controlled movements, breathing in for 1 circle and out for the next.

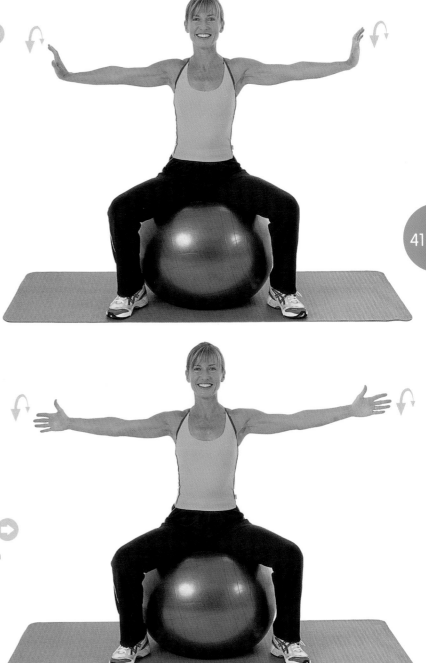

TRAINER'S TIPS

❶ Relax your shoulders and think of lengthening your arms out sideways. Do not take your arms behind the line of your shoulders.

❷ Caution! If you feel any prickling in your fingers – STOP.

41

Start as above, but now face your palms forwards and point your thumbs towards the ceiling. Lengthen your fingertips out to the side and perform 8 circles forwards and then 8 circles backwards to complete 1 set. Breathe in for 1 circle and out for the next.

Reach for the Sky

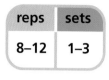

reps	sets
8–12	1–3

This shoulder press is a challenging exercise. Your whole shoulder area will be strengthened, your upper back and the backs of your arms toned and sculpted. Your stomach muscles will work at maintaining stability in your spine, making this a truly effective movement for enhancing posture and balance.

Select suitable weights (see page 11). With a dumb-bell in each hand, sit upright on the ball with your spine in a neutral position (see page 16). Position your knees over your feet. Maintain this upright posture. Bend your arms at 90 degrees and bring your elbows level with your shoulders. Your palms should face forwards. This is the start position.

Breathing out, push the dumb-bells upwards, raising your arms above your head. Keep a slight bend in your elbows to avoid them locking. Look straight ahead. Then, breathing in, lower your arms back to the start position; avoid dropping your elbows as you do so.

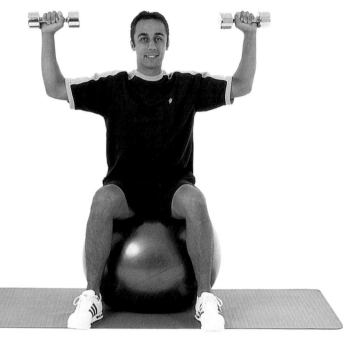

TRAINER'S TIPS

❶ Pull your navel in towards your spine to maintain good posture and anchor your body.

❷ If you feel unstable, widen your knees so that they point slightly outwards and are positioned over your toes.

Front Lifts

reps	sets
8–12	1–3

This movement focuses on strengthening and shaping the fronts of the shoulders and also provides definition to the fronts of the arms. Combine this with other shoulder exercises to achieve balanced, toned and shapely shoulders.

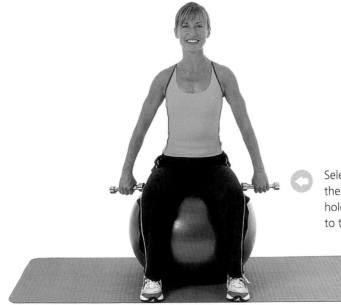

Select suitable weights (see page 11). Sit upright on the ball, with your knees positioned over your feet, holding a dumb-bell in each hand. Bring your arms to the sides of the ball, palms facing backwards.

43

TRAINER'S TIPS
1. Keep your navel pulled in towards your spine to support your back.
2. Breathe out as you raise the dumb-bells, breathe in as you lower them.
3. Avoid leaning backwards when you lift the dumb-bells. Lift no higher than shoulder height.

With a slight bend in your elbows, slowly raise both the dumb-bells in front of you up to shoulder level. Hold for a second, then lower to the start position.

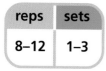

Rear Shoulder Lifts

reps	sets
8–12	1–3

Focusing on the backs of the shoulders, these lifts quickly tone and eliminate flab from that hard-to-reach area that everyone can see apart from you! Rear lifts also help to sculpt and define the backs of the arms, another area prone to losing muscle tone.

TRAINER'S TIPS

❶ Imagine, from the side, your back making a long diagonal line from your 'tailbone' to your head. Make sure you keep your head and neck in line with your spine.

❷ Avoid lifting your chin by looking slightly downwards and forwards.

❸ **Caution!** If you generally suffer any neck weakness or pain, perform this exercise without using weights.

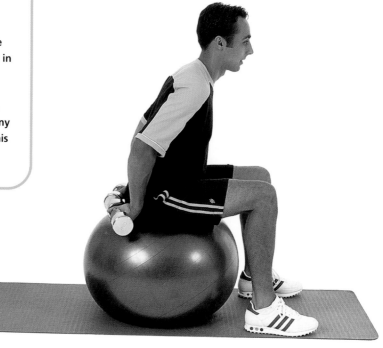

⬆ Select suitable weights (see page 11) and sit upright on the ball. Keep your knees parallel and over your feet. Pull your navel in towards your spine and lean forward slightly from your hips. Lengthen your back and keep it straight. Hold the weights behind you in line with your body; do not rest them on the ball.

⬅ Lift and raise the dumb-bells behind you, breathing out on the raise and in as you lower. Gently squeeze your shoulder blades at the top of the movement, hold for a second, then return slowly to the start position.

44

Wing Beats

reps	sets
8–12	1

This toning exercise sculpts the mid-shoulder area, giving the tops of your arms and shoulders shape and definition. Performing this movement on the ball improves your balance, while your stomach muscles work hard to support your back.

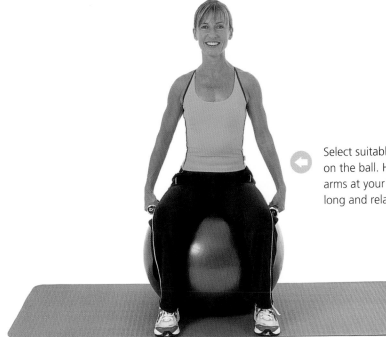

Select suitable weights (see page 11) and sit upright on the ball. Hold a dumb-bell in each hand with your arms at your sides, palms facing in. Keep your neck long and relax your shoulders.

Slowly raise your arms out to the side to shoulder level, with slightly bent elbows. Your palms should now face down. Hold for a second, then slowly lower your arms to the start position.

TRAINER'S TIPS
1. Avoid locking your elbows, and lift your arms no higher than shoulder level.
2. Keep your navel pulled in towards your spine.
3. Breathe out as you lift your arms, breathe in as you lower them.

45

Shoulder Shapers

reps	sets
8–12	1–3

The group of small muscles at the back of each shoulder play an important role in overall posture; they also rotate the arms. These muscles need to be strengthened to pull the shoulders back and help guard against injury. This simple exercise helps to prevent rounded shoulders.

Select lighter weights for this exercise (see page 11). Sit on the ball and hold a weight in each hand. Position your knees over your feet. Pull your navel in towards your spine to stabilize your back. Bring your elbows close to your sides at waist level, palms facing up.

Rotate the dumb-bells outwards, keeping your elbows close to your sides. Bring them back to the start position.

TRAINER'S TIPS
1 Breathe out as you rotate the dumb-bells outwards, breathe in as you return to the start position.
2 Keep your elbows close to your sides.
3 Avoid flexing your wrists.
4 Keep your navel pulled in towards your spine throughout.

Flabby-Arm Farewell

reps	sets
8–12	1–3

This exercise sculpts the triceps muscles at the backs of the arms. The backs of the arms are one of the first areas to lose shape – particularly on women, who unfortunately accumulate fat here. This movement tones and defines the triceps, with the bonus of toning the backs of the legs, buttocks and stomach muscles, all of which work to stabilize your body on the ball.

Select suitable weights (see pages 11). Start from the Walkaway position (see pages 34–35), lying with your head, neck and shoulders supported on the ball. Place your knees over your feet. Pull your navel in towards your spine and lift your buttocks. Hold the dumb-bells above your head, with slightly bent elbows.

47

Bend and pivot from your elbows, keeping your upper arms still, and, breathing in, slowly lower the dumb-bells towards your ears. Then breathe out as you push back upwards until your arms are nearly straight. Avoid locking your elbows.

TRAINER'S TIPS

1 Keep your elbows parallel and close to your head. Pivot from your elbows for correct technique.
2 Your hips must stay still to maintain good body alignment.

Overhead Triceps Press

reps	sets
8–12	1–3

This exercise targets the backs of the arms and provides a seated alternative to the Flabby-Arm Farewell (see page 47). It also challenges your stomach and back muscles, helping to improve core stability and balance.

Select one dumb-bell of suitable weight (see page 11). Sit upright on the ball with your spine in a neutral position (see page 16). Position your knees over your heels. Hold the dumb-bell behind your head: your elbow must be level with your head. Use the opposite hand to hold the triceps area gently and help you maintain good arm alignment.

Breathe out as you slowly push the weight upwards. Keep your elbow close to your head and avoid locking your elbow as you extend your arm. Hold for a second, then breathe in as you return to the start position.

48

TRAINER'S TIPS
1. Pull your navel in towards your spine throughout to avoid arching your back.
2. Bend from your elbow, keeping your upper arm still.
3. Use slow, controlled movements.
4. Do not allow your elbow to drift outwards.

Drop Dips

reps	sets
8–12	1–3

This is a more demanding exercise that uses your own body weight with the ball. It works the triceps muscles at the backs of your arms and challenges your shoulders, building strength and stability in these often weaker muscles.

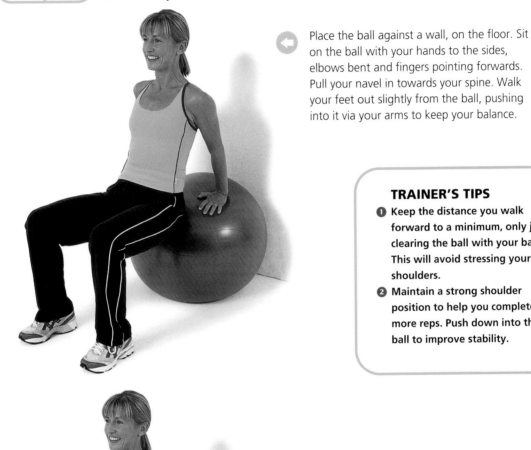

Place the ball against a wall, on the floor. Sit on the ball with your hands to the sides, elbows bent and fingers pointing forwards. Pull your navel in towards your spine. Walk your feet out slightly from the ball, pushing into it via your arms to keep your balance.

TRAINER'S TIPS

❶ Keep the distance you walk forward to a minimum, only just clearing the ball with your back. This will avoid stressing your shoulders.

❷ Maintain a strong shoulder position to help you complete more reps. Push down into the ball to improve stability.

49

Breathe in and bend your elbows to a comfortable angle without losing control. Breathe out as you straighten your elbows and avoid locking them.

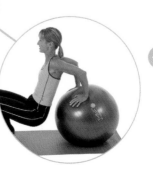

Megachallenge!
To increase the intensity, perform Drop Dips without bracing the ball against a wall.

Biceps Curl

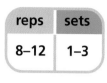

reps	sets
8–12	1–3

This excellent exercise works the biceps muscles at the front of your upper arms, developing lean definition and giving shape to this area. Using the ball here provides support for your back, which is particularly beneficial for anyone who suffers from back discomfort. Developing strength in your upper arms means you can take everyday activities in your stride.

Select suitable weights (see page 11). Place the ball against a wall, nestling it comfortably in the small of your back. Hold the dumb-bells with palms facing forwards and arms by your sides. Keep your knees slightly bent.

Breathe out and keep your elbows close to your body as you lift the dumb-bells up to your shoulders. Squeeze your biceps at the end of the curl, then slowly lower back to the start position, breathing in as you do so.

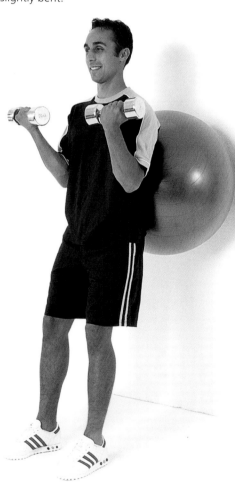

TRAINER'S TIPS

❶ Look straight ahead to keep your head aligned with your spine.

❷ Pull your navel in towards your spine to maintain good posture.

❸ Keep your movements slow and controlled – never let momentum carry you through.

Hammer Curl

reps	sets
8–12	1–3

This variation on the basic Biceps Curl is a valuable exercise because it works on toning and defining the outer part of your upper arms. It will help your arms look leaner and longer, more sculpted. Used as part of a balanced upper-body workout, the Hammer Curl produces excellent results.

Select suitable weights (see page 11). Place the ball between you and the wall, nestling it in the small of your back. Hold a weight in each hand with your elbows close to your sides, palms facing in. Keep your back straight and your knees slightly bent.

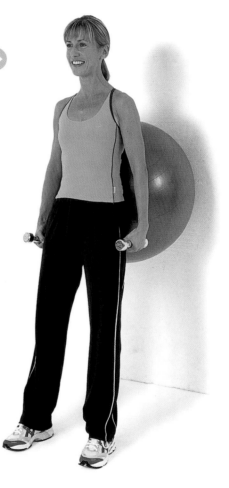

Keeping your elbows close to your sides, lift the dumb-bells towards your shoulders. Squeeze your biceps at the end of the curl, then lower to the start position. Breathe out as you lift, breathe in as you lower.

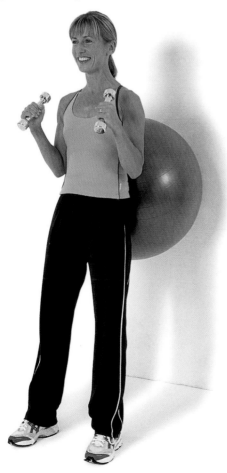

51

TRAINER'S TIPS
1. Pull your navel in towards your spine throughout.
2. Avoid locking your elbows.
3. Keep your back straight.

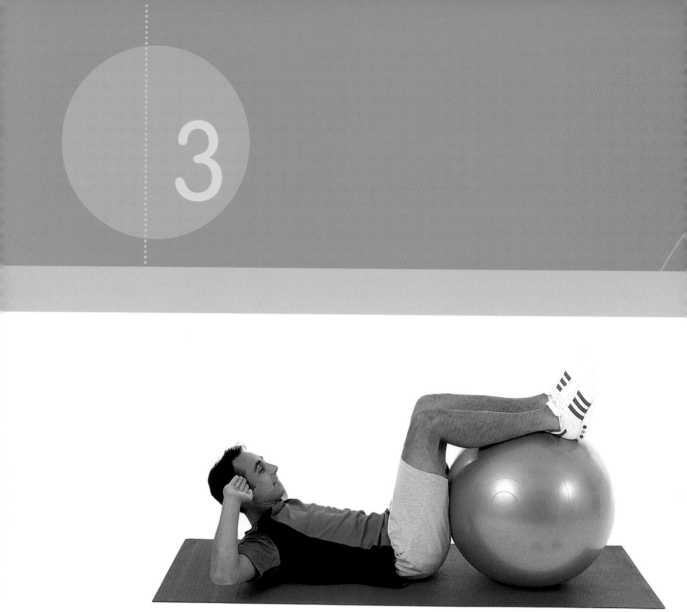

abdominals and back

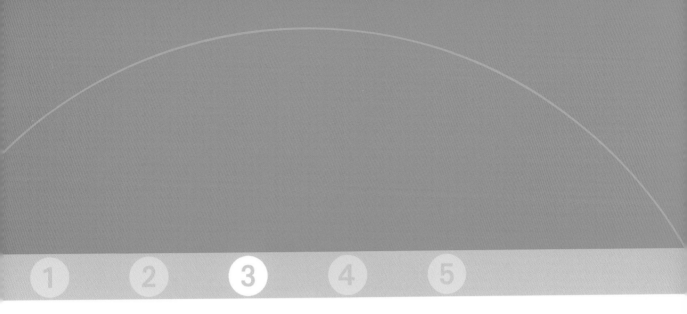

If you want a toned, defined mid-section you need to target the muscles that act like a corset on the whole abdominal area and you need to be disciplined about training them. Exercising with the ball can achieve results more quickly than other types of workout and is very effective in enhancing your core stability, by conditioning the deep-seated muscles that support your back. A strong back will provide you with a secure base for all types of activity.

When you work out on the ball you have to use your postural muscles to hold it steady in a variety of positions, making abdominal work on the ball incredibly effective. The exercises provided here target your core muscles in a completely balanced programme that is suitable for everyone.

It is up to you to make the habits of 'pulling your navel in towards your spine' and 'pulling up tall' part of your everyday life. Eventually, by combining abdominal work on the ball with consciously holding yourself upright, your stomach muscles will hold themselves in without you having to do anything!

The back programme complements the abdominal workout to give you a strong, flexible and healthy spine, as well as muscular balance. It will also improve your posture, helping to eliminate round shoulders and/or a hollow back. By working your stomach and back muscles in a balanced programme, you will create a strong centre that helps to eliminate back pain and makes you look taller and feel younger.

53

Supaman

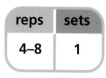

reps	sets
4–8	1

This is an effective movement that helps to establish muscular strength and control in your back, lower stomach and buttock muscles. It also focuses on balancing the muscles from the upper back down to the hip area. Start with the basic version (steps 1 and 2 below) and move on to the intermediate (step 3) and more advanced (step 4) versions only when you find the previous stage easy.

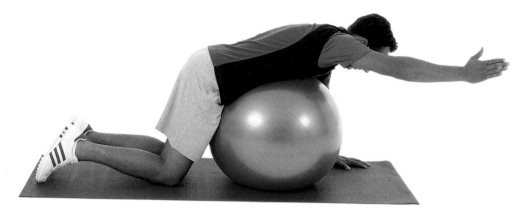

⬆ Lie over the ball on all fours, with hands and knees positioned on the floor. Pull your navel in towards your spine and keep your head in line with your spine. Lift your right arm straight in front of you, without lifting your shoulder blades upwards towards your ears. Hold for up to 5 seconds, then lower to the start position. Repeat on the other side.

TRAINER'S TIPS

❶ Keep your toes near the floor when learning this move.

❷ Avoid lifting your leg above hip level as this will make your back arch and will stress your spine.

❸ Only progress to the next level when you find these two exercises easy.

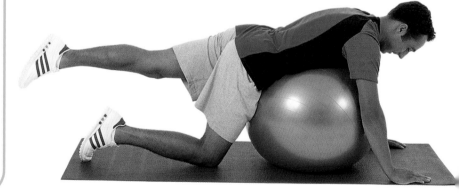

⬆ From the same start position, slowly straighten and extend your left leg out behind you. Imagine there is a straight line from your toes to your ears. Use your buttock muscles to lift your leg and avoid sideways hip movement. Hold for up to 5 seconds, then lower to the start position. Repeat on the other side.

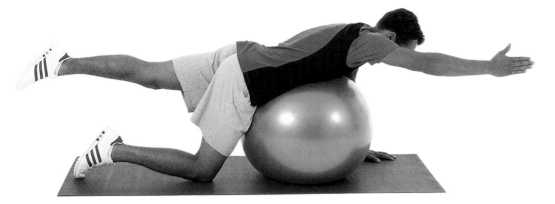

For the intermediate version, lie on the ball as before. Using the opposite arm to the lifting leg, combine the previous arm and leg lifts by raising both together. Lift the leg only to hip level and raise the opposite arm only to ear level. Hold for up to 5 seconds, then lower to the start position. Repeat on the other side.

For the advanced version, extend one leg behind you without using your arms for support or balance; place your arms at your sides. Pull your navel in towards your spine and keep your head in line. Hold for up to 5 seconds, then lower to the start position. Repeat on the other side.

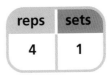

reps	sets
4	1

Megachallenge!
Progress to lifting both arms, with one leg extending out behind you. Hold for up to 5 seconds, then lower to the start position. Repeat on the other side.

TRAINER'S TIPS
1. Avoid sideways movements in your hips.
2. Avoid letting your head drop. Do not look up, as this will strain neck muscles.
3. Keep your supporting elbow bent.

Body Wave

reps	sets
5–8	1

A superb core exercise, the Body Wave prepares your spine for the work ahead by mobilizing your back and releasing tension. This movement strengthens the back and buttocks while activating the hamstrings. It will help you to control each part of your back and uses your abdominal muscles to stabilize you.

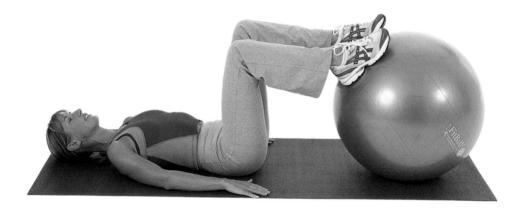

TRAINER'S TIPS

❶ Picture each section of your spine as you roll up. As you roll down, imagine your spine is a car tyre making an imprint of its tread in your mat.

❷ The backs of your legs work hard in this exercise, so you may need to start off with just a couple of reps and increase the number gradually.

❸ **Caution!** Do not push up too high, as this will put undue strain on your neck.

⬆ Lie on your back with the soles of your feet resting on the ball. Your knees should be bent at 90 degrees. Breathe in to prepare.

⬇ Breathing out, pull your navel in towards your spine and lift and curve your hips off the floor. Pressing your feet in to the ball, roll up slowly through your spine until you reach the upper mid-back area. Hold this position for a second while breathing in, then slowly lower through your spine as you breathe out. Make sure your movements are slow and controlled and keep the ball still.

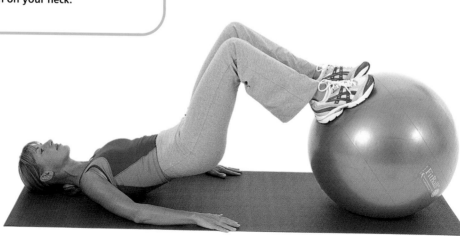

Prone Ball Row

reps	sets
8–12	1–3

This is a first-class strengthening exercise for the neck and mid-back area that also benefits postural muscles. This movement focuses on weaker areas of your body that are often the cause of injury. For the less fit or those with back discomfort, it can be practised without weights. When choosing weights, use light dumb-bells to begin with (see page 11).

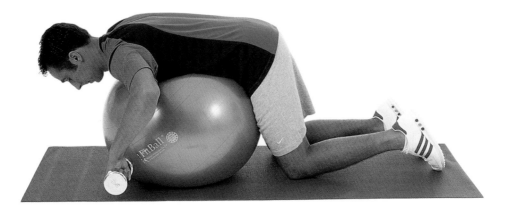

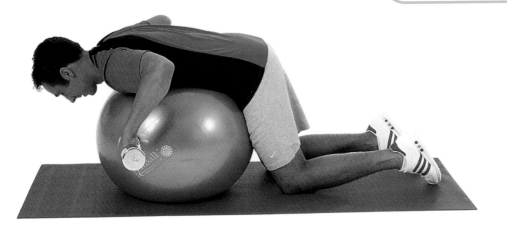

⬆ Lie on the ball with your body weight supported. Bend your knees and extend your arms forwards slightly to the floor; your hands are underneath your shoulders. Hold the dumb-bells in an over-hand grip. Breathe in to prepare.

⬇ Breathe out as you lift the dumb-bells upwards, leading with your elbows in a rowing movement, then lower to the start position.

TRAINER'S TIPS

❶ Pull your navel in towards your spine to support your back throughout.

❷ Keep your neck lengthened and look down towards the floor to maintain the correct neck alignment.

❸ If you are not using dumb-bells, imagine you are pulling your elbows upwards in a slow rowing action.

57

Lean Lats

reps	sets
8–12	1–3

This exercise strengthens and tones the back muscles that shape the outer mid-back area. These large muscles in the back are sometimes difficult to tone effectively. This movement on the ball works to balance them, with the bonus of giving your back a good shape because of the large area they cover. For best results, select a slightly heavier weight (see page 11).

TRAINER'S TIPS

❶ Pull your navel in towards your spine to hold you firmly on the ball and prevent your back from arching.

❷ Try not to over-extend your arms.

❸ Use slow, controlled movements.

❹ Breathe in as you extend your arms backwards, breathe out as you bring them back to eye level.

⬇ Lie back on the ball with your head, neck, shoulders and back supported. Hold one large dumb-bell in both hands, starting with the weight above your head at eye level. Keep your elbows slightly bent.

⬇ Slowly extend your arm and lower the dumb-bell behind your head until you feel a stretch through your outer mid-back area, and then return the dumb-bell to the start position.

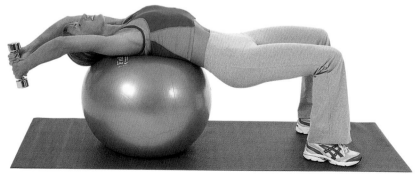

58

Shoulder Glider

reps	sets
8–12	1–3

This superb exercise tones and strengthens the mid-back area, making it particularly useful for people who play racquet sports, golf, hockey and bowls. A well-toned back is an asset, looks great and gives balance to toned stomach muscles to provide perfect posture. Attention to technique is vital: your stomach is called on to support your spine and keeps your torso stable, while you work your shoulder blades and contract your back muscles.

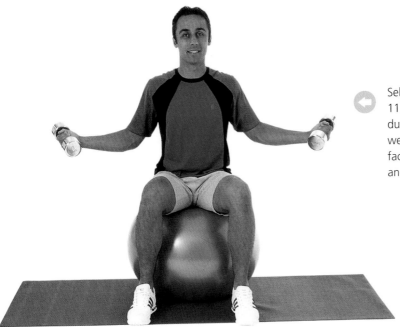

Select suitable weights (see page 11). Sit upright on the ball with a dumb-bell in each hand. Hold the weights out to the side, palms facing up. Keep your elbows bent and slightly behind your waistline.

TRAINER'S TIPS
❶ Keep your navel pulled in towards your spine throughout.
❷ Imagine squeezing an orange between your shoulder blades.
❸ Avoid hunching your shoulders.

Bring your elbows in to your sides. Squeeze your shoulder blades together as your elbows move in and down. Release back to the start position.

Body Bow

reps	sets
8–12	1–3

This simple torso extension is an easy exercise for strengthening and toning your back and neck muscles. It's ideal for making everyday tasks such as gardening, lifting young children and housework much less arduous. This is a less-demanding back exercise than the Human Cannonball (see opposite).

TRAINER'S TIPS

❶ Avoid clasping your hands behind your head as this will put pressure on your neck.
❷ Pull your navel in towards your spine as you lift.
❸ Do not lift too high: your torso should make a diagonal line when seen from the side.
❹ Keep your chin tucked in to maintain good neck alignment.

Lie over the ball on your stomach, with your knees bent on the floor. Touch your hands to the sides of your head. Keep your eyeline towards the floor. Breathe in to prepare.

Breathe out as you lift your chest off the ball. Keep your shoulders and neck in line with your back as you extend your body. Lower to the start position.

Human Cannonball

reps	sets
8–12	1–3

This fabulous exercise uses the ball to support your body while strengthening your lower back and buttock muscles, which will help you achieve core stability and correct posture. Strengthening your lower back can help prevent injuries. To perform this exercise safely and well, make sure your feet are on a non-slip surface; otherwise, brace them against a wall.

TRAINER'S TIPS
① Keep the movement small.
② Lengthen outwards from the top of your head.
③ **Caution!** Avoid tipping your head up – keep your chin tucked in.

61

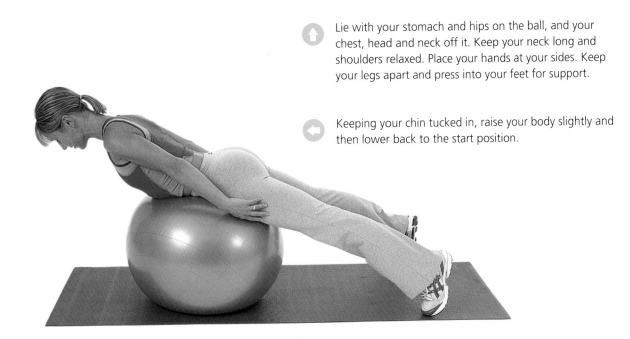

Lie with your stomach and hips on the ball, and your chest, head and neck off it. Keep your neck long and shoulders relaxed. Place your hands at your sides. Keep your legs apart and press into your feet for support.

Keeping your chin tucked in, raise your body slightly and then lower back to the start position.

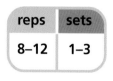

Up, Up and Away

reps	sets
8–12	1–3

This exercise targets the arms, back and neck muscles for improved strength and endurance. Your posture will improve tremendously: you will walk and stand without slouching, making you appear taller and slimmer. Everyday tasks like lifting and carrying will be far less tiring.

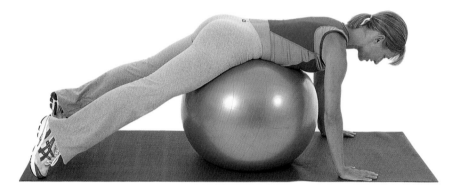

Lie with your stomach and hips on the ball. Extend your legs, pushing into the floor with the balls of your feet. Place your hands under your shoulders to support your upper-body weight. Your head must be in line with your spine. Breathe in to prepare.

62

TRAINER'S TIPS

❶ Pull your navel in towards your spine as you raise your torso.
❷ Avoid lifting your chin as this will put strain on your neck.
❸ Caution! Lift your body until it is in a straight line – do not arch your back upwards.

Breathe out, lifting and reaching upwards. Raise your torso and arms as you lengthen and extend out through your fingertips. Keep your head between your arms with your chin tucked in. Lower to the start position.

Aeroplane

reps	sets
8–12	1–3

The Aeroplane helps your back muscles learn how to balance movement. This demanding exercise challenges your buttocks to support your spine. Your stomach muscles also have to work hard to stabilize you throughout the rotational movements.

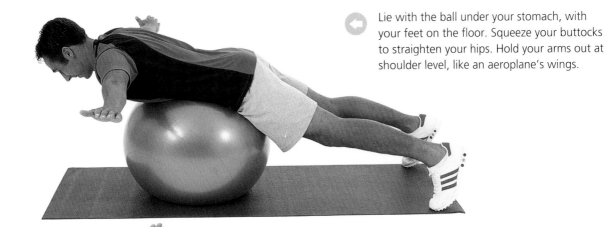

Lie with the ball under your stomach, with your feet on the floor. Squeeze your buttocks to straighten your hips. Hold your arms out at shoulder level, like an aeroplane's wings.

Keep stabilized on the ball as you turn your upper body so that your right hand touches the floor. Use your stomach muscles to turn yourself back to the start position. This is 1 rep. Now repeat on the other side.

63

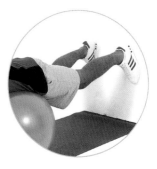

Megachallenge!
For high-flyers, perform the Aeroplane with your feet against a wall, positioned slightly lower than hip level.

TRAINER'S TIPS
1. Pull your navel in towards your spine and keep your shoulders relaxed.
2. Focus on using your buttocks to avoid over-using your back muscles.
3. **Caution!** Do not turn your head too far to each side as you rotate your body.

Huggaball

reps	sets
8–12	1

This exercise not only trains your stomach muscles but is also an excellent way of learning how to establish a good breathing technique. The ball compels your spine to shape around it as you develop awareness of, and focus on, the deepest layers of your stomach muscles. This enables you to concentrate on expanding your lungs into the sides and back of your ribs. This wonderfully calm exercise is excellent for reducing stress and inducing relaxation.

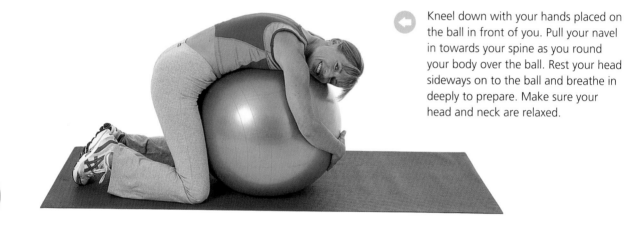

Kneel down with your hands placed on the ball in front of you. Pull your navel in towards your spine as you round your body over the ball. Rest your head sideways on to the ball and breathe in deeply to prepare. Make sure your head and neck are relaxed.

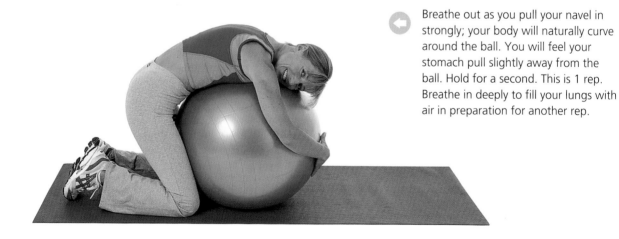

Breathe out as you pull your navel in strongly; your body will naturally curve around the ball. You will feel your stomach pull slightly away from the ball. Hold for a second. This is 1 rep. Breathe in deeply to fill your lungs with air in preparation for another rep.

Ab-Alert

reps	sets
8–12	1

The Ab-Alert makes you conscious of how your stomach muscles respond to the demands placed on them, especially when movements are performed from a variety of directions. This fundamental exercise will increase your awareness of the muscles that form a major part of your core strength and is especially appropriate for anyone new to exercise training.

Lie on your back with your knees bent and feet hip-width apart. Place your hands on each side of the ball and hold it up at chest level, with your elbows slightly bent. Pull your navel in towards your spine and straighten your arms to lift the ball upwards.

Slowly move the ball behind your head. You will feel your spine arching off the floor – you must now pull in your navel even more and consciously narrow the gap between your ribs and your hips. Return the ball to the start position.

TRAINER'S TIPS

❶ Perform the movements slowly for maximum benefit.
❷ For extra intensity, start by holding the ball with your arms extended over your right shoulder and then take the ball diagonally across to your left hip. Repeat on the opposite side.

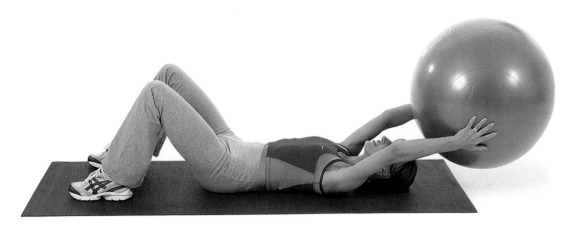

Basic Ab-Fabs

reps	sets
8–12	1–3

This floor-based work is a good starting point for anyone new to stomach exercises. It provides an excellent preparation for strengthening your upper abdominal area in a simple-to-learn movement. Basic Ab-Fabs will speed you towards a firmer, flatter stomach and more defined musculature.

Lie with your legs on the ball. The ball should be near your buttocks, with your hips and knees bent at 90 degrees. Touch your hands to your head. Breathe in to prepare.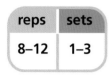

Breathe out as you raise your head and shoulders off the floor; imagine an orange between your chin and your chest. As you lift up, pull your navel in towards your spine and slide your ribs towards your hips. Hold for a second, then breathe in and lower to the start position.

TRAINER'S TIPS
❶ Keep your shoulders relaxed – do not tense up.
❷ Avoid pulling on your neck.

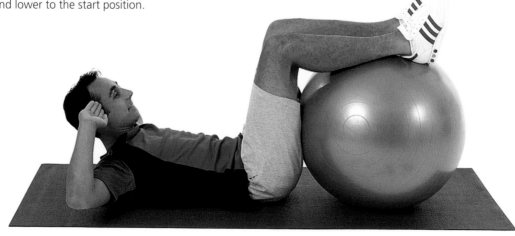

Basic Ab-Fab Twists

reps	sets
8–12	1–3

This is the floor-based version of the Ab-Fab Twists (see page 69), designed to get you going before tackling the ball-based exercise. It will suit the less fit and anyone who wants to tone and shape their waist area. The twisting movement works the oblique muscles that run down the sides of your torso from the ribs to the hips, producing a narrower waist.

TRAINER'S TIPS
1 Breathe out as you lift up, breathe in as you lower.
2 Pull your navel in towards your spine as you lift up.
3 Keep your elbows open.
4 Avoid pulling on your neck.

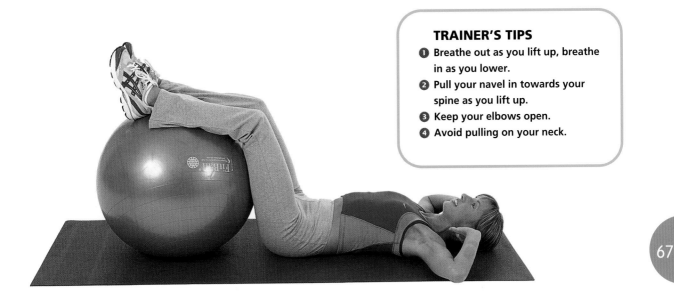

Lie on your back with your legs on the ball. The ball should be close to your buttocks, with your hips and knees bent at 90 degrees. Place your hands lightly behind your head without clasping them together.

Raise your head and shoulders from the floor and rotate your upper body, starting from the right shoulder. Imagine holding an orange under your chin, and try to bring your ribs over to the opposite hipbone. Hold for a second, then lower to the start position. Perform the required number of reps on the same side before changing to the other side.

Abs-olutely Fabulous

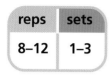

reps	sets
8–12	1–3

This is a very effective way of training your stomach muscles. The ball supports the hollow of your lower back, which allows your abdominal muscles to work through a larger range of motion than is possible in floor-based abdominal exercises. Other muscles also have to work hard to maintain your balance on the ball.

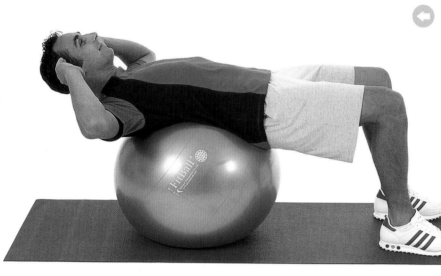

Sit on the ball, then walk your feet out until the ball is supporting your lower back. If you feel uncomfortable, drop your hips to sit lower. Your feet should be shoulder-width apart, with your knees over your heels. Place your hands lightly behind your head. Imagine holding an orange under your chin.

TRAINER'S TIPS
1 Breathe out as you lift up, breathe in as you lower.
2 Pull your navel in towards your spine throughout.
3 Make sure the small of your back is supported by the ball.
4 This is a controlled raise – do not curl right up.

Lift your shoulders and slide your ribs down towards your hips, contracting your stomach muscles. Hold for a second, then lower to the start position.

Ab-Fab Twists

reps	sets
8–12	1–3

This stomach exercise produces amazing results, working the abdominal muscles far more efficiently than traditional floor-based work. The ball promotes a greater range of movement, allowing maximum isolation of the abdominals, while other muscles are recruited to stabilize you. You will achieve a firm, flat stomach and toned waistline in no time.

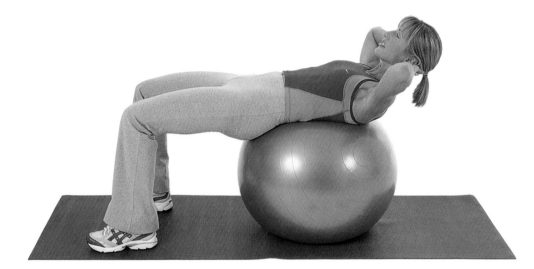

Sit on the ball and walk your feet out so that your lower back is supported by the ball. Position your feet shoulder-width apart, with knees over heels. Place your hands behind your head and imagine holding an orange under your chin. Pull your navel in towards your spine.

Breathing out, lift your shoulders and rotate your upper body, starting from the right shoulder. Try to bring your ribs over to the opposite hipbone. Hold for a second, then breathe in and return to the start. Repeat on the other side.

TRAINER'S TIPS
1. Keep your elbows open, and avoid pulling on your neck.
2. When this exercise becomes easy, try performing 8–12 reps on one side, followed by 8–12 reps on the other.

Waist Whittler

reps	sets
8–12	1–3

This exercise targets the oblique muscles at the sides of your waist and makes your stomach and back muscles (your 'core' strength) work together to maintain balance and control throughout the movement. Regular practice will trim your waistline and improve your posture.

Brace your feet in a stride position against a step or wall. Position the ball under the side of your body at hip level. Pull your navel in as far as you can and place your fingertips on your temples. Keep your elbows back and squeeze your shoulder blades together.

Slowly lower and arch your body sideways over the ball. Keep your abdominal muscles firmly contracted as you slowly raise back to the start position.

70

TRAINER'S TIPS

1. Breathe in as you lower, breathe out as you lift up.
2. Keep your head in line with your spine and avoid pulling on your neck.
3. Use slow, controlled movements throughout.

Reverse Curls

reps	sets
8–12	1–3

This effective exercise concentrates on the lower area of the abdominal muscles, where the most stubborn of 'spare tyres' resides. Much stomach work focuses on the central and upper abdominals, whereas Reverse Curls get down to the lower part of your stomach. You will really feel this area working hard!

> **TRAINER'S TIPS**
> ❶ Keep your neck and shoulders as relaxed as possible.
> ❷ Avoid pushing against the floor with your arms – that's cheating!
> ❸ Avoid swinging your legs – that's also cheating!

Lie on your back, gripping the ball firmly under your calves. Rest your arms at your sides, palms facing up. Using your heels, hitch the ball into the backs of your legs.

Pulling your navel in towards your spine, slowly raise the ball from the floor and hold for a second, breathing out as you do so. Then relax your stomach muscles, breathe in and lower the ball towards the floor, without letting it actually touch the floor. This completes one rep.

71

Off-Side Rolls

reps	sets
8–12	1–3

This is an easy combination exercise that strengthens your oblique (waist) muscles while also toning your hips and legs. It is suitable for every level of fitness, but particularly those who are less fit or the overweight exerciser.

Lie on your back and rest your heels on the top of the ball. Pull your navel in towards your spine and look up to the ceiling. Your palms face down with your arms at your sides.

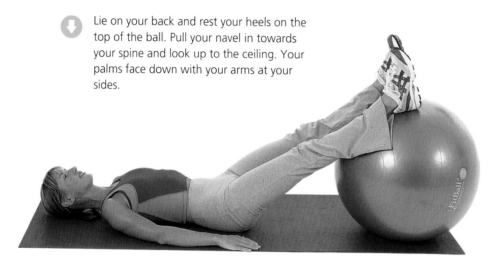

Slowly roll the ball from one side to the other, maintaining control of it by using your stomach muscles. Concentrate on feeling your oblique abdominal muscles working. Keep your legs straight.

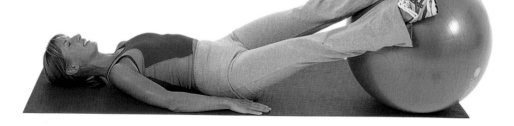

TRAINER'S TIPS
❶ Keep all your movements smooth and controlled.
❷ Avoid your back lifting off the floor by keeping your navel pulled in firmly throughout.

Knees Up

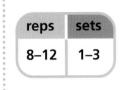

reps	sets
8–12	1–3

This is a refreshingly different way to exercise your stomach muscles, adding variety to your workout. It strengthens your stomach and arms, and the movement of your legs forces your abdominal muscles into action. It's a great ball exercise that works several muscle groups to strengthen, tone and sculpt.

Start from the Wheelbarrow position (see page 32), with your thighs on the ball, navel pulled in towards your spine, and shoulders over your hands.

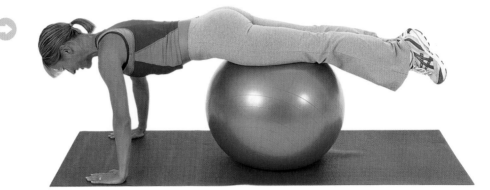

TRAINER'S TIPS
❶ Keep your navel pulled in firmly towards your spine to stabilize your back.
❷ Keep ball movements in a straight line, as if on a railway track.
❸ **Caution!** Avoid looking up or you may strain your neck.

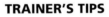

73

Bend your legs and draw your knees inwards. Keep your arms stable.

Continue drawing your knees up towards your chest, until you reach the position shown. Return to the start position, using your stomach muscles to maintain control.

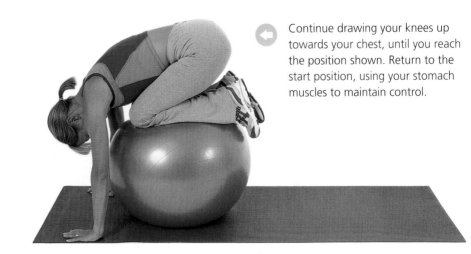

Ab-Activator

reps	sets
1	1

With this exercise, your stomach, back and shoulder muscles all work as a unit. Hold the position only for as long as you feel comfortable and build up your strength gradually. With all versions of the Ab-Activator, always start by kneeling down with the ball in front of your knees and placing your hands on the ball. This will ensure a safe and stable start.

From the start position, push the ball slightly away from you and lean forward, placing your bent elbows on the ball with your hands clasped together. Pull your navel in towards your spine. Pull the ball back slightly, making sure that only your shoulders move, and hold until you tire.

Extended Arms Ab-Activator

reps	sets
1	1

This is a more intense version to which you can progress as soon as the standard Ab-Activator becomes easy.

Assume the start position, with your elbows pushed into the ball and hands clasped together. Now push further forwards, so that your arms extend more and hold for a second. Pull the ball back in towards you and hold this position until you tire. Keep your back in a straight line from your shoulders to your hips.

TRAINER'S TIP
Caution! If you have any history of shoulder problems, consult a physiotherapist before performing these Ab-Activator exercises.

Off-Toes Ab-Activator

reps	sets
1	1

Attempt this version only when you find the other two variations easy.

Assume the original start position. Concentrate hard and slowly straighten your body as you push up on to your toes. Push down into the ball through your elbows.

Move the ball away slightly by moving your arms forwards. If your back dips, pull your arms back slightly towards you. Pull your navel in towards your spine to maintain a straight line from the back of your head to your knees. Now pull the ball towards you and hold until you tire.

TRAINER'S TIPS
1 Keep your navel pulled firmly in towards your spine throughout to avoid hollowing out your spine
2 **Caution!** Listen to your body – if it's uncomfortable, STOP!

Kickstart

reps	sets
4	1–3

This is an intense abdominal workout suitable for the advanced exerciser. Kickstart places demands on your core stability and challenges your stomach strength, balance and coordination skills. Learn this exercise one stage at a time. Only progress when a stage is no longer testing your strength and balance. You will need a clear wall space to perform this exercise.

Place the ball against the wall. Lean forwards on to the ball with your elbows bent and hands clasped together. Straighten your body, pull your navel in towards your spine and balance on the balls of your feet.

Maintaining a neutral spine position (see page 16), slowly bring your right knee up towards the ball, breathing out. Then extend your leg back to the start position, breathing in. Do this 4 times with the right leg, then repeat with the left leg. This completes 1 set.

TRAINER'S TIPS

❶ Push down strongly into the ball through your elbows to maintain stability and prevent your shoulders lifting.

❷ Keep your navel pulled in firmly towards your spine to maintain correct spine alignment.

No-Wall Kickstart

reps	sets
4	1–2

This really intensive version of the Kickstart relies on your own strength and balance to anchor the ball – without the wall!

Assume the same start position but without the supporting wall.

TRAINER'S TIPS
1 Maintain straight back alignment throughout.
2 Avoid rounding your back, lifting your shoulders or over-extending your arms.
3 When extending your leg back again, do not lift it too high – this will lead to poor alignment.

77

This time bring your knee closer to your stomach while drawing the ball inwards using your elbows. Breathe out as you do so.

Pull your navel in towards your spine and breathe in as you extend your right leg backwards. Keep the ball controlled, so that your elbows move forwards slightly but under control. Do this 4 times with the right leg, then repeat with the left leg. This completes 1 set.

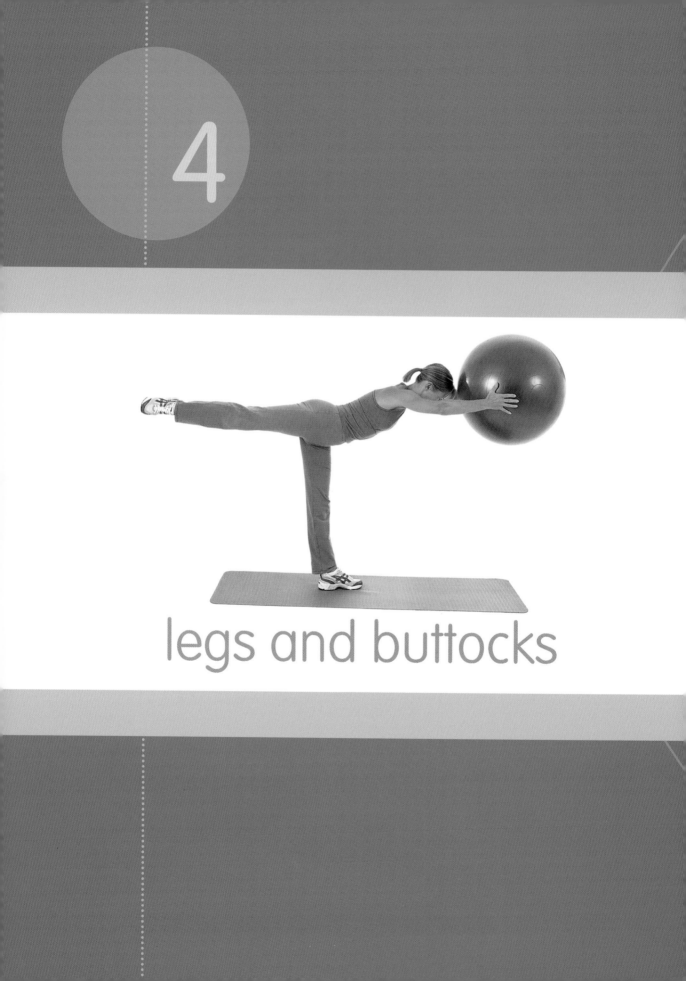

4

legs and buttocks

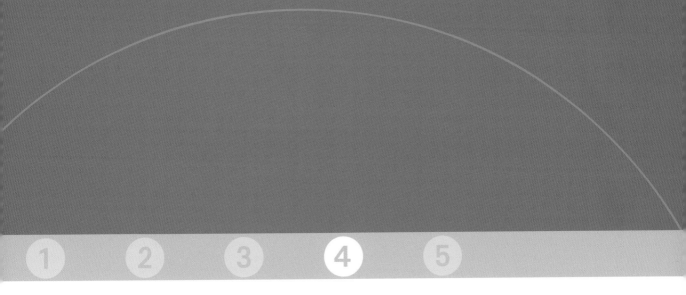

Strong, toned legs and buttocks look good and are essential for a healthy, balanced body. The leg exercises in this chapter cater for all fitness levels and are designed to sculpt and tone the weaker muscles at the backs of the thighs; create definition and lift between the buttocks and the backs of the legs; shape the fronts of the thighs without any bulking; and condition the inner thighs.

Firm, toned buttocks are something we would all like. The buttocks are responsible for dynamic movements and guard against back and knee injuries. The exercises here will firm and tone your buttock muscles without overbuilding them.

Be clear about your aims. Extensions and rotations work on shaping your buttocks for a firm, round appearance: choose exercises like

Wall Crawl, Ball Frog and Abductor Rotator. To reduce buttock size, concentrate on low-intensity exercises like the Elevator, Ball Drag, Rollover and Seesaw, performing them more often. Also include plenty of aerobic exercise.

To tackle cellulite, combine these leg and buttocks exercises with eating a healthy diet (see page 11); drinking at least 8 glasses of water daily; and brushing your skin regularly with a natural bristle brush to improve circulation and help reduce any mottled appearance.

Following this balanced leg and buttocks workout will help you to achieve your aim of lissom legs and a refined behind! By combining these with the routines in chapters 2 and 3, you'll soon have a perfectly firm, toned body.

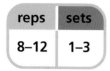

Pennyfarthing

reps	sets
8–12	1–3

This wonderful routine shapes and tones the backs of the legs (hamstrings). It coordinates the hamstrings and buttocks in a push-and-pull action that produces maximum results. The Pennyfarthing is suitable for all fitness levels.

Lie on your back and rest your right leg on the ball. Bend your left leg and place the sole against the ball. Rest your arms at your sides, palms facing down.

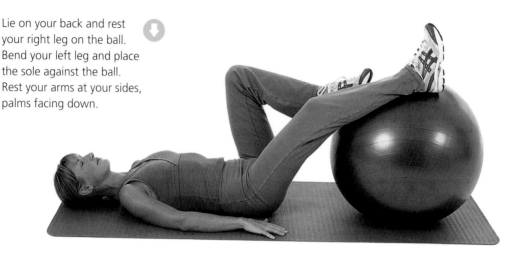

80

Keep your torso stable by pulling your navel in towards your spine. Press your right heel down and pull the ball towards you, at the same time pushing the ball away from you with your left foot. The ball should remain still. Maintain this balanced pressure for about 3 seconds, then release. Do this 8–12 times on one leg, then change to the other.

TRAINER'S TIPS
❶ Protect your back by pulling your navel in towards your spine throughout.
❷ To intensify the exercise, increase the distance between the ball and your buttocks.
❸ Keep the ball still by balancing the push-and-pull action of your legs.
❹ Make sure your buttocks lift up only slightly from the floor during the exercise.

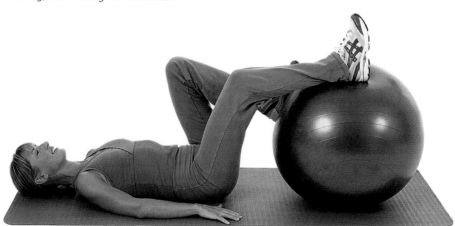

Elevator

reps	sets
8–12	1–3

Ideal for strengthening and sculpting the buttocks and backs of the thighs, this exercise also improves stability in your torso and increases the range of movement in your hips. The Elevator prepares you for the more demanding leg work to come.

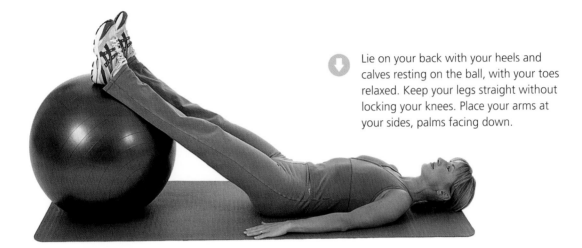

Lie on your back with your heels and calves resting on the ball, with your toes relaxed. Keep your legs straight without locking your knees. Place your arms at your sides, palms facing down.

Tighten your buttocks and slowly lift your hips off the floor, as you push your heels down into the ball. Hold for a second, then slowly lower your hips to the floor.

81

TRAINER'S TIPS
❶ Keep your navel pulled in towards your spine as you lift your hips off the floor.
❷ Visualize pushing down into your feet to keep the intensity in your legs, not your back.
❸ Keep the ball steady – don't let it wander!
❹ For less intensity, keep the ball closer to your buttocks.

Megachallenge!
Perform the exercise as before but with your arms raised towards the ceiling. This challenges your balance, as you cannot use your arms to stabilize you.

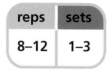

Ball Drag

reps	sets
8–12	1–3

The Ball Drag challenges the whole lower body and trunk. It is a truly multipurpose exercise that targets the buttocks, backs of the legs, calves, lower back, pelvic floor and core stabilizing muscles. Improving strength and balance in all these areas makes the Ball Drag a really effective and versatile exercise.

> **TRAINER'S TIPS**
> ❶ Avoid starting with the ball too far away from you or you will lose it.
> ❷ When lifting your hips, push down into your feet otherwise your back may arch.

82

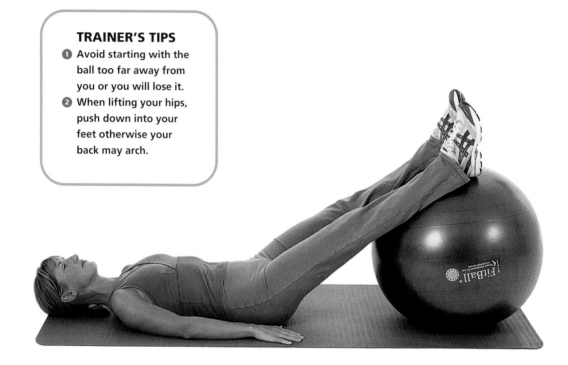

🔼 Lie on the floor with your legs straight and your heels and calves resting on the ball. Place your arms at your sides, palms facing down, and relax your neck and shoulders.

🔽 Tighten your buttocks, pull your navel in towards your spine and lift your hips upwards until your legs and shoulders form a diagonal line.

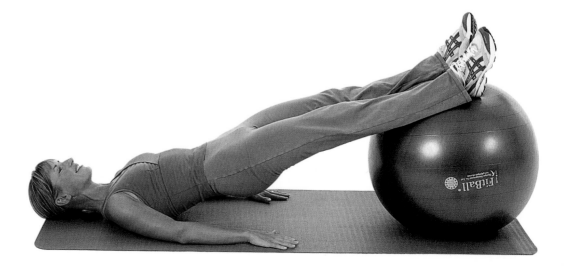

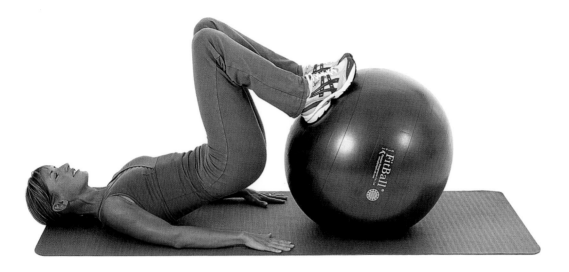

↑ Push down into the ball through your feet and pull the ball in towards your buttocks as far as you can. Keep your buttocks lifted. You will feel the muscles working from your calves through to your buttocks.

↓ Push into the ball and slowly straighten out your legs again, keeping the ball steady. Lower your hips back to the start position.

83

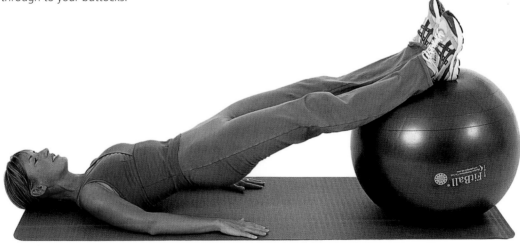

TRAINER'S TIPS
1. Keep your ball movements in a straight line, as if it is on a railway track.
2. Keep your neck and shoulders as relaxed as you can to avoid unnecessary tension.

Single-Leg Ball Drag

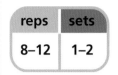

reps	sets
8–12	1–2

This is a more demanding version of the Ball Drag (see pages 82–83). The emphasis is on the back of the working leg. Only attempt this when you can perform 2 sets of 12 reps of the standard Ball Drag with ease.

◄ Lie on your back with your right heel and calf resting on the ball. Put your left leg in the air, slightly bent at the knee. This leg must stay anchored in this position.

84

TRAINER'S TIPS

❶ Avoid swinging your lifted leg to and fro, otherwise you will lose stability and compromise your technique.

❷ Push into the foot on the ball to prevent your back from arching as you lift your hips.

❸ Always stretch the backs of your legs after every set of this intense exercise. (See Scissor Stretch on page 118.)

▼ Push down into the ball with your right heel and tighten your buttocks as you lift your hips off the floor. Keep your navel pulled in towards your spine.

Push into your right heel and pull the ball in towards your buttocks as far as you can. Keep your buttocks lifted. You should be able to feel the muscles all along the back of your right leg working hard.

Push your heel into the ball as you straighten your right leg and lower your buttocks to return to the start position. Perform the required number of reps, then work the left leg.

TRAINER'S TIPS
1. To enhance stability, keep your navel pulled in towards your spine.
2. Keep ball movements in a straight line, as if it is on a railway track.
3. Keep your hands, shoulders and neck relaxed throughout.

85

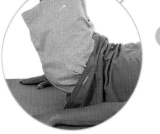

Megachallenge!
To add extra intensity to the exercise, do not lower your buttocks to the floor between reps.

Ball Frog

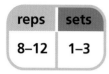

reps	sets
8–12	1–3

This is a version of the Ball Drag (see pages 82–83). Working the hamstrings and calves, it gives an extra challenge to the deep layers of muscle in the buttocks. It also tones the inner thighs, and will really test your balance.

Lie on your back with your heels and calves resting on the ball. Place your arms at your sides, palms facing down.

Tighten your buttocks and slowly lift your hips off the floor as you push down through your feet.

As you do so, pull the ball in towards your buttocks as far as you can and hold for a second.

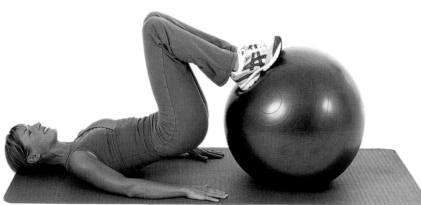

TRAINER'S TIPS
❶ Pull your navel in towards your spine throughout to stabilize your back.
❷ Avoid pushing up from your hips as this will force your lower back to arch.
❸ **Caution!** If you suffer from sciatica do not attempt this exercise.

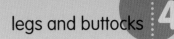
Now gently squeeze the outsides of your buttocks and turn your knees out – imagine a frog position!

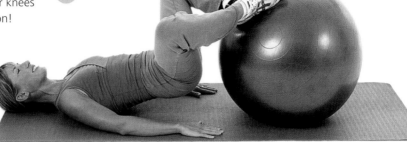

Tighten your outer buttocks and squeeze your inner thighs as you bring your knees back together. Now push down into the ball through your feet and straighten out your legs.

87

TRAINER'S TIPS

1. Remember to squeeze your buttock muscles on the 'turn out' movement.
2. Pull your navel in towards your spine to improve your balance.
3. Keep movements slow and controlled – good technique is crucial for success.

Keep your buttocks contracted and your hips lifted. Your legs will now be parallel and straight. Turn your toes out while keeping your heels together, keeping your pelvis square. Bring the toes back to a straight position, then lower your hips to the floor.

Wall Crawl

reps	sets
8–12	1–3

The squat is one of the most effective exercises for the legs, buttocks and lower back. The Wall Crawl intensifies the exercise because the ball supports your back, allowing your buttocks and thighs to work harder.

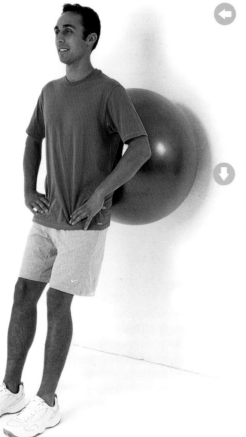

Place the ball against the wall between your mid- and lower back. Keep your back straight, with hands on hips for balance. Pull your navel in towards your spine. Your feet should be shoulder-width apart with your hips level, and your knees slightly bent and in line with your ankles.

Slowly roll your body down until your thighs are parallel with the floor. Then slowly roll back up to the start position. Focus your thoughts on your thigh muscles, which will help to maximize the effect of the exercise.

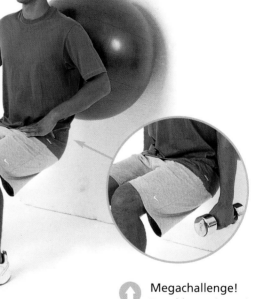

TRAINER'S TIPS

❶ For a less intense version, stop when your thighs are at 45 degrees to the floor, then return to the start position.

❷ **Caution!** Do not take your hips lower than the level of your knees, as this will put excessive and damaging strain on your knee joints.

Megachallenge!
To add extra intensity, repeat the standard Wall Crawl while holding dumb-bells throughout.

Static Wall Crawl

reps	sets
1	1

This is a challenging variation on the Wall Crawl that will really develop your leg strength.

Use the Wall Crawl start position, but place your hands on your thighs. Slowly roll down until your thighs are parallel with the floor. Hold for as long as you can, then slowly roll back to the start position.

Single-Leg Wall Crawl

reps	sets
8–12	1–2

Move on to this version when the Wall Crawl no longer challenges you. It will develop your leg strength but will also enhance balance and co-ordination.

Use the Wall Crawl start position. Lift one leg off the floor, bending at the knee so that your thigh is parallel with the floor. Now bend your standing leg to a half-squat position, keeping the supporting knee in line with your ankle. Return to the start position. Perform the required number of reps on each leg. This completes 1 set.

TRAINER'S TIP
To prevent the standing knee rolling inwards, tighten the buttock muscle on the supporting side.

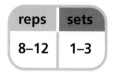

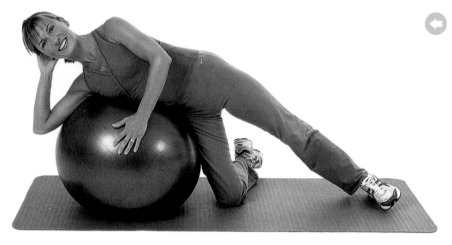

Abductor Constructor

reps	sets
8–12	1–3

This clever outer-thigh and hip exercise really reaches its target! It challenges your core muscles to hold your body firm as you arch sideways into the ball. At the same time, your outer thighs and hips are toned and strengthened.

Kneel at the side of the ball with it close to your right thigh. Lean over the ball, pulling it tightly into your waist and hip. Rest your head on your right hand and hold the ball with your left hand. Extend your left leg sideways, with your knee and your toes facing forwards.

Lift your left leg slowly and lengthen it away from you. Raise it no higher than your hip, then slowly return to the start position. Perform the required number of reps, then change to the other leg for the required number of reps, to complete 1 set.

TRAINER'S TIPS

1 Do not allow your body weight to sink into your supporting hip, otherwise you will tire rapidly.

2 Keep pulling your navel in towards your spine throughout – if your stomach sags so will everything else!

Megachallenge!

On the last leg raise of each set, keep your leg lifted and point your toes. Now move your leg in 8 small circles, first clockwise then anticlockwise, lengthening outwards before lowering.

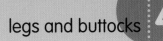

Abductor Rotator

reps	sets
8–12	1–2

A more advanced and demanding variation of the Abductor Constructor (see opposite), this exercise not only targets the hips and thighs but also shapes the buttocks beautifully. It requires good technique to ensure you gain full benefit from this challenging movement, so pay attention to your body position throughout.

Adopt the start position as for the Abductor Constructor. Pull your navel in towards your spine. Lift your right leg slowly no higher than your hip and lengthen it away from you.

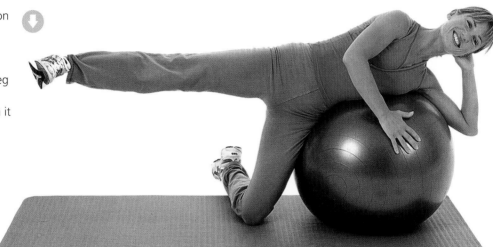

Keeping your leg at hip height, rotate it outwards slightly, from the hip joint, while squeezing your buttocks. Now rotate your leg to face forwards, then slowly lower to the start position. Perform the required number of reps on each leg. This completes 1 set.

TRAINER'S TIPS
1. Keep the knee of the raised leg slightly bent to avoid stressing the joints.
2. Do not allow your hips to twist as you rotate your leg.
3. Pull your navel in towards your spine.

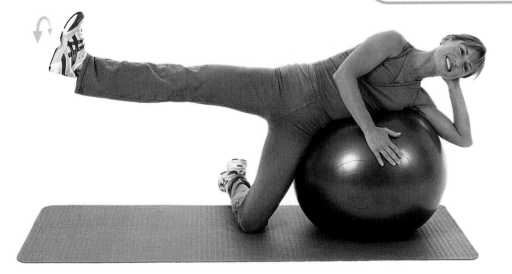

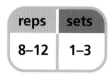
Inner-Thigh Eraser

reps	sets
8–12	1–3

This intense exercise works the adductor muscles hard while engaging the thighs and buttocks. These inner-thigh muscles are some of the most underused in the body and are quite difficult to train effectively. The Inner-Thigh Eraser will shape, tighten and tone this area. It is very important to keep your knees bent and to build up the number of reps gradually.

Lie on your back with your legs raised and the ball between your bent knees. You may need to hold the ball with your hands to keep it in position. Gently squeeze the ball with your inner thighs and knees. Hold for a second, then release and repeat. When starting, do as many reps as is comfortable and build up gradually to the target number.

TRAINER'S TIPS
1. Pull your navel in towards your spine to prevent your back arching.
2. As the exercise becomes easier, try holding the squeeze for several seconds.
3. To perform the Megachallenge with good technique, keep your knees slightly bent.

Megachallenge!
To add extra intensity, place the ball between your ankles and your calves, then squeeze and release as before.

Bellows

reps	sets
8–12	1–3

This simple-to-perform exercise tones and firms the inner thighs beautifully. Flabby, weak inner thighs do not receive the attention they should because they can be difficult muscles to target successfully. You will feel this movement isolating and working your adductor muscles. Some people find it better to deflate the ball slightly for this exercise.

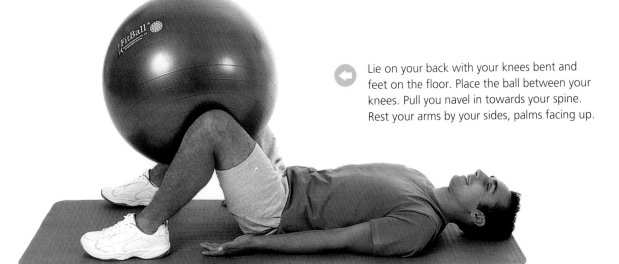

Lie on your back with your knees bent and feet on the floor. Place the ball between your knees. Pull you navel in towards your spine. Rest your arms by your sides, palms facing up.

TRAINER'S TIPS
1. As you squeeze the ball, keep your navel pulled in towards your spine to avoid arching your back.
2. Speed up or slow down the tempo of the squeezes to vary the intensity of the exercise, and hold the squeeze for longer to maximize the effect.

Gently and firmly squeeze the ball between your knees and inner thighs. Hold for a second, then release.

Lift and Balance

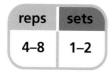

reps	sets
4–8	1–2

This is a good wake-up exercise for a sluggish central nervous system and will improve your balance and proprioceptive skills (the body's ability to contract muscles so that posture and balance are maintained, and actions are smooth and co-ordinated). Lift and Balance requires a high level of concentration and will help you to develop good coordination. It will train your body to avoid falls and improve your reactions to unexpected dangers.

Stand with your feet hip-width apart and hold the ball in front of your legs. Pull your navel in towards your spine. Relax and consciously drop your shoulders.

Slowly lift your left knee, drawing your foot up the side of your right calf until your thigh is parallel to the floor. At the same time, raise the ball with your arms extended at chest height. Try and avoid locking the supporting leg.

TRAINER'S TIP

It will help your balance if you concentrate on keeping your body weight travelling centrally through your supporting leg and down into your heel.

Keeping your left knee at the same height, extend your leg in front of you while you lift the ball above your head. Keep your eye focused on something at eye level to avoid wobbling. Slowly bring your left leg back to the bent-knee position, and lower the ball to your thighs as you return your left foot to the floor. Do the required number of reps, then change to the other leg.

Seesaw

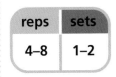

reps	sets
4–8	1–2

This demanding exercise is a bit different and enormously effective. It will improve strength in your lower back, abdominals, buttocks and thighs by using the ball to provide resistance for the upper body. Practising the Seesaw will enhance your balance, coordination and proprioceptive skills, training your body to cope with unexpected physical dangers.

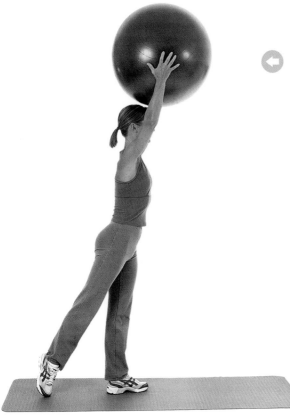

Start with your right leg behind you lightly touching the floor and hold the ball above your head. Lift up out of your hips, pull your navel in towards your spine and look straight ahead.

Slowly lift your right leg off the floor, lengthening out behind you; at the same time, reach outwards and lower the ball. The ideal position to achieve is a straight line from the ball to your toes that is parallel to the floor. At first you may only be able to balance at an angle to the floor – this is fine, provided you always imagine yourself as the 'plank' on the seesaw and maintain a straight alignment from toes to ball. Perform the required reps before changing to the other leg.

95

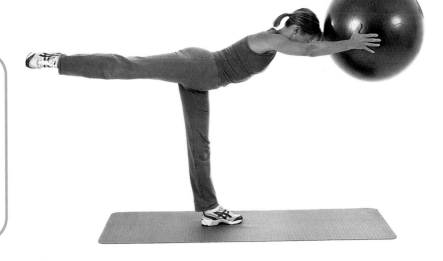

TRAINER'S TIPS
❶ Keep your arms and legs at the same level.
❷ Reaching out in both directions will help you to balance.
❸ Wobbling is quite normal – but you will improve with practice.

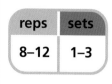

Wall Slide

reps	sets
8–12	1–3

This exercise will strengthen your knees and hip muscles, gently stretch your hamstrings and increase your range of motion. It's a good movement to practise at any fitness level and is ideal for anyone with weak knees or hips, making it particularly suitable for mature exercisers.

Lie on your back with both knees bent. Place the ball against the wall and put your right foot against it. Your left foot should be flat on the floor and your arms relaxed at your sides, palms facing up.

Slowly extend your right leg and roll the ball up the wall slightly. Lower your right leg and the ball back to the start position. Perform the required number of reps, then change to the other leg.

TRAINER'S TIPS

❶ Keep your neck and shoulders relaxed.
❷ Pull your navel in towards your spine throughout to avoid your back arching.
❸ Use slow, controlled movements throughout.

Megachallenge!
This variation provides an extra challenge and double the benefits! Perform the standard Wall Slide, but this time with both legs on the ball at the same time.

Knee Lifts

reps	sets
8–12	1–3

This straightforward exercise works the hip flexors, activates the lower abdominal muscles and tones the thighs. Here the ball encourages balance and coordination and also makes this routine suitable for the more mature exerciser. Progress to the Megachallenge once standard Knee Lifts no longer test your ability.

Sit upright on the ball and position your knees over your heels. Focus directly ahead of you and rest your hands on your hips. Pull your navel in towards your spine and tighten your buttock muscles to maintain stability.

97

TRAINER'S TIPS

❶ This looks simple, but balancing on the ball requires concentration. Think about pulling up and lengthening from the top of your head.

❷ Use your stomach muscles to help you balance.

Lift up your left knee and hold for 3 seconds, then lower back to the start position. Repeat with your right leg.

Megachallenge!

This advanced version will shape and tone the fronts of your thighs. This time, as you lift your knee extend your leg straight out in front of you at hip height.

Rollover

reps	sets
8–12	1–3

A more advanced leg-strengthening exercise, the Rollover also helps to mobilise your upper mid-back, activates your abdominals and shapes your arms. Perform this exercise slowly with control in order to achieve sound technique and good alignment, both vital in gaining maximum results.

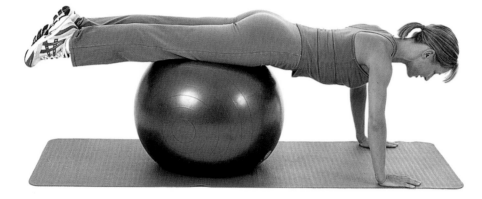

Start in the Wheelbarrow position (see page 32). Your shoulders should be over your hands, and the fronts of your upper thighs should rest on the ball with your legs straight. Use your stomach muscles to stabilize your spine.

Slowly roll the ball sideways under your left thigh, stopping when the outer side of your thigh is in contact with the ball. Your right leg simultaneously extends upwards off the ball and allow your elbows to bend slightly. Keep looking at the floor; your head must stay in line with your shoulders. Return to the start position, lowering your right leg under control. Repeat with the other leg.

TRAINER'S TIPS
1 Avoid lifting your leg too high otherwise your back will arch, leading to poor body alignment.
2 **Caution!** Do not turn to look at your lifted leg – you may strain your neck.

Heel Hoists

reps	sets
8–12	1–3

This simple exercise, suitable for all fitness levels, concentrates on strengthening the ankles and improving their mobility. It is great for sportspeople at risk of ankle damage, such as footballers, and is also of huge benefit to older people, for whom ankle weakness is a common cause of falls. It also works the calf muscles.

Sit upright on the ball, pulling your navel in towards your spine. Keep your shoulders open and relaxed, and rest your hands on your hips. Your knees should be positioned over your heels.

99

TRAINER'S TIPS

❶ To increase the benefit, try speeding up the tempo of the hoists, lightly tapping the floor on the return.

❷ The fronts of your shins and ankles can be further improved by doing Toe Hoists, lifting your toes up towards the shins instead of lifting your heels.

Megachallenge!
Intensify the Heel Hoists by holding dumb-bells on the fronts of your thighs.

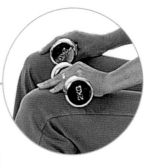

Slowly lift your heels off the floor, hold for a second, then lower them back to the floor.

Thigh Trimmer

reps	sets
8–12	1–3

This is a bargain of an exercise with a basketful of benefits! It will strengthen and tone both the inner and the outer thighs and engage the lower abdominal area. Your stomach and back are forced to work hard together to stabilize you, while your thighs are trimmed, toned and streamlined.

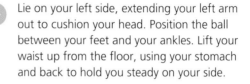

Lie on your left side, extending your left arm out to cushion your head. Position the ball between your feet and your ankles. Lift your waist up from the floor, using your stomach and back to hold you steady on your side.

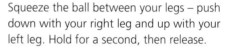

Squeeze the ball between your legs – push down with your right leg and up with your left leg. Hold for a second, then release.

TRAINER'S TIPS

1 Pull your navel in towards your spine throughout.
2 If your neck is uncomfortable, place a small cushion between your arm and your head.
3 Keep your upper shoulder relaxed.
4 Do not let your waist drop back towards the floor.

Swiveller

reps	sets
8–12	1–3

This exercise will challenge your coordination. You have to synchronize and control your movements, along with correct positioning. The rewards for all this juggling are strong, toned inner and outer thighs, hip muscles and abdominals, plus increased range of motion in your hips. Well worth the effort!

Lying on your back, bend your knees up and lift both legs towards the ceiling. Place the ball centrally between your feet and ankles. Apply gentle pressure to hold the ball securely in position.

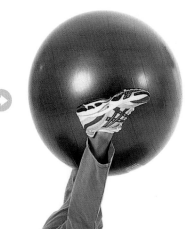

TRAINER'S TIPS

1. Pull your navel in towards your spine throughout to avoid arching your back off the floor.
2. Start with 5–6 reps and build up gradually.
3. Co-ordination is crucial – you will keep dropping the ball if one leg works harder than the other!

101

Slowly rotate the ball between your feet. Move your right foot towards you until your heel is pressing against the ball; at the same time, move your left foot away from you so that your instep presses into the ball. Now reverse the rotation, so that your right foot is now further away from you and your left foot is closer to you.

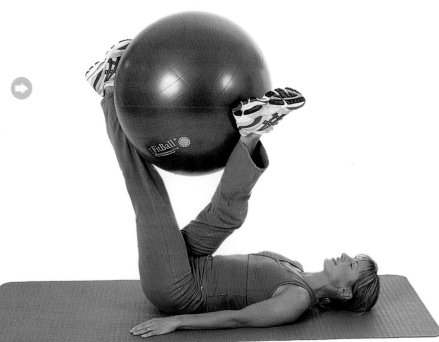

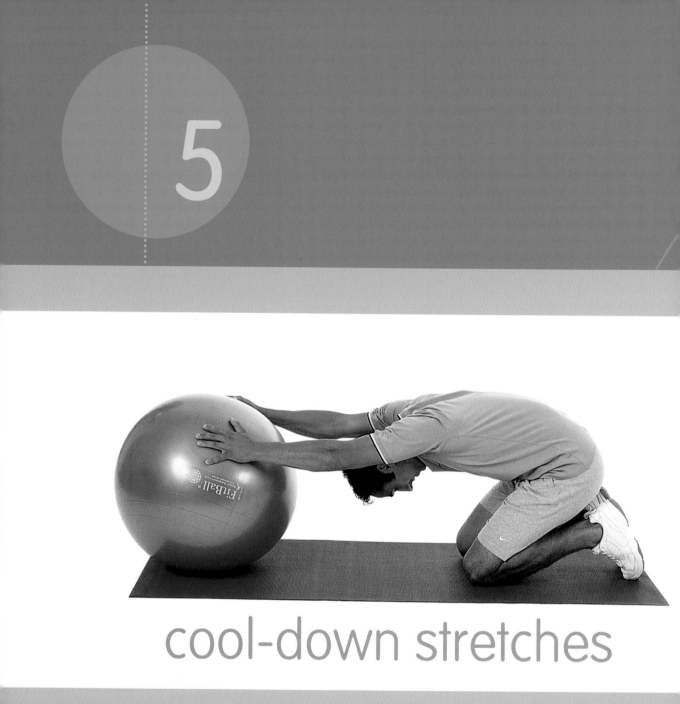

cool-down stretches

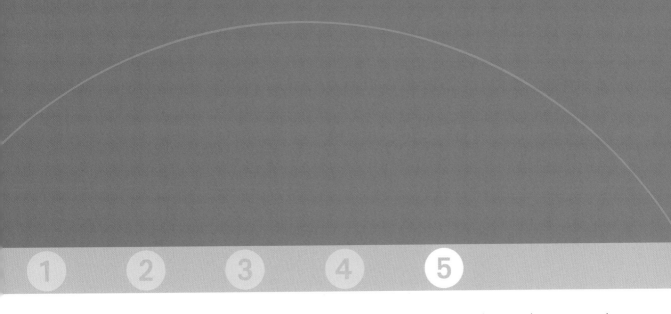

Active people lead full lives: they enjoy better health, high levels of confidence and are generally happy. We currently have a huge problem dealing with the effects of sedentary lifestyles, and one of the most important gaps to bridge between an active and a sedentary life is to become more flexible. Stretching is vital.

Regular stretching helps to improve your mobility and flexibility, particularly as you get older, and reduces your chances of injury. Stretching also requires you to centre your thoughts on individual parts of the body, increasing your ability to clear your mind and focus on detail.

The exercises in this chapter can be used equally well as a stretching programme on their own or as a cool-down after exercising. Stretching after exercise is vital, because the muscles are receptive when warm: it will help both to lengthen your muscles and to disperse any lactic acid that forms during your exercise session.

Stretching helps you to relate movement to breathing, which is fundamental to disciplines such as yoga and other relaxation techniques. Regular stretching also helps you to detox by stimulating better circulation.

Stretching is not competitive – only stretch as far as you are comfortable. Take the exercises slowly, easing gently into each stretch. Focus on 'feeling' your muscles, which will encourage a calm, more responsive body. Stretching is a natural tranquillizer and will induce a serene sense of well-being – so relax and enjoy.

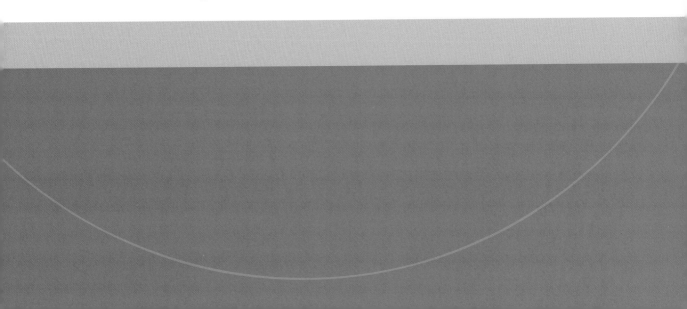

Archway

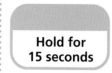

Hold for 15 seconds

This is a lovely relaxing movement that opens up the chest area and stretches out the shoulder muscles. Tension held in the chest can lead to poor posture. Use the Archway as a cool-down stretch after exercising or to unwind and release tension.

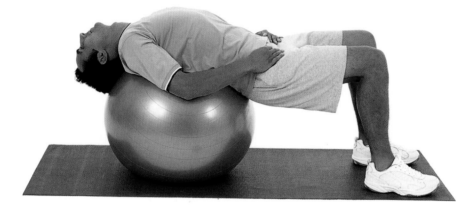

TRAINER'S TIPS
❶ If the stretch feels too intense, try lowering your hips towards the floor.
❷ Keep your breathing slow and controlled.

⬆ Sit upright on the ball with your hands on your hips and your navel pulled in towards your spine. Walk your feet out, allowing your back to mould into the ball.

⬇ Resting your back, shoulders and head on the ball, reach your arms over your head, palms facing up. Feel the wonderful soothing stretch in your chest muscles.

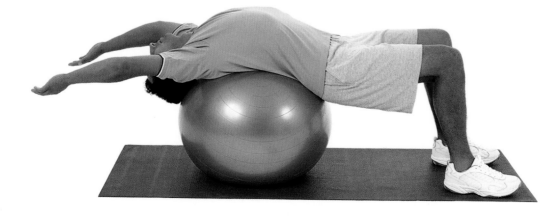

Tension Tamer

reps	sets
6–8	1

Shrugs are a classic exercise for releasing tension and strain in the shoulders and neck. It is surprising how much these areas suffer in everyday activities, bent over a desk, sitting at a computer and behind the wheel of a car, or just carrying children or shopping. Tension Tamer really de-stresses and frees up a knotty, aching neck and shoulders.

Sit on the ball with your knees over your feet. Focus on relaxing while gently pulling your navel in towards your spine. Rest your hands at your sides and look straight ahead.

105

TRAINER'S TIPS
1. You may find you gain full benefit by doing only 3 or 4 shrugs.
2. Visualizing the tension flowing out with each shrug really does help.
3. Allow your arms to hang loose and relaxed.

Draw your shoulders up towards your ears as far as you can manage comfortably. Hold for 2–3 seconds, then drop your shoulders and relax.

Crescent Stretch

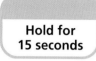

Hold for 15 seconds

This graceful, relaxing stretch lengthens the whole torso from the shoulder all the way down to the hip. The ball provides a perfect base on which to stretch out your sides. Ideal for easing out any tension in your body, it is also a fantastic stretch after exercise. Overall, a superb general relaxation movement to refresh you.

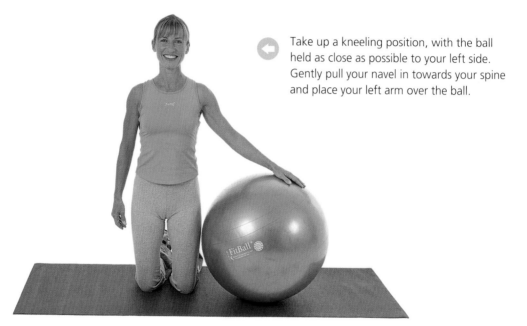

Take up a kneeling position, with the ball held as close as possible to your left side. Gently pull your navel in towards your spine and place your left arm over the ball.

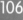
TRAINER'S TIPS
① Keep your head and neck relaxed and look straight ahead.
② Feel and enjoy the stretch all along the side of your body.

Stretch your right arm upwards and arch your body sideways over the ball, reaching over your head with your right arm and extending out with the left. Your left leg remains bent while your right leg straightens out to the side. Hold, then repeat on the opposite side.

Banana Bend

Hold for 15 seconds

A sitting-on-the-ball variation of the Crescent Stretch (see opposite), this version stretches the length of the torso. It achieves a great stretch from the shoulder through to the hip and is excellent for relieving muscular tension in the body, particularly after exercising the stomach and back.

Sit up tall on the ball and gently pull your navel in towards your spine. Rest your left hand lightly on your left thigh and hold your right arm above your head.

107

Reach up and over sideways with your right arm until you feel a comfortable stretch along the right side of your torso. As you curve over, move your left arm across the opposite hip. Hold, then repeat on the other side.

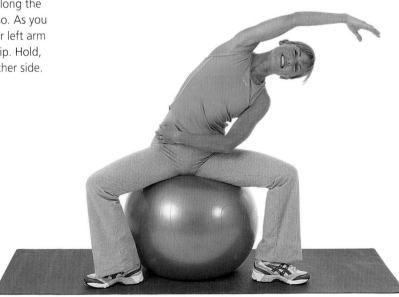

TRAINER'S TIPS

❶ Breathe in as you lift up, breathe out as you reach over, then breathe slowly and evenly as you hold the stretch.

❷ Keep central on the ball – do not allow the ball to shift to the side.

Torso Stretch

Hold for 10 to 15 seconds

Although this is a gentle movement to perform, it is a highly effective way to release tension across the whole back area: the rotational movement stretches and relaxes muscles that are often hard to reach. After a strenuous workout or a hard day at work, the Torso Stretch will leave you feeling revived and refreshed.

Sit on the ball with your knees together and over your feet. Place your left hand on the outside of your right thigh, palm facing out. Put your right hand on the ball behind you with the palm facing down.

Lift up out of your hips. Pressing your left hand against your right thigh, rotate to your right. Turn your head and upper body as far round as is comfortable without twisting your hips. Hold, then return to the start position. Repeat on the other side.

TRAINER'S TIPS

❶ Keep your navel pulled firmly in towards your spine throughout.
❷ Avoid sinking into your hips as you turn round.
❸ Visualize the top of your head spiralling up to the ceiling as you rotate.

Lower-Spine Soother

Hold for 30 seconds

This stretch is an all-time favourite because it feels so good! You really feel your back relaxing, and you can adapt your position to achieve the best possible stretch for you. This is an excellent stretch after an exercise session, but use it every day and it will help alleviate aching and stiffness in your back.

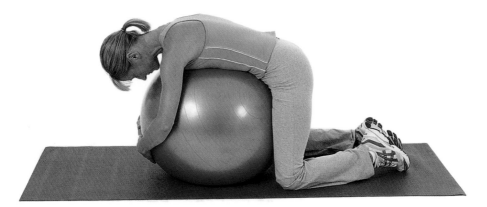

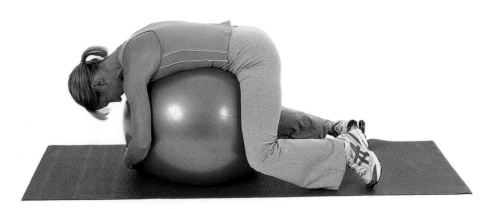

↑ Start by kneeling in front of the ball, pulling it close to your thighs. Lean into the ball on your stomach and bend your knees to the sides of the ball.

↓ Now relax forwards over the ball and hug it close to your body, so that your spine rounds over the shape of the ball. Hold.

TRAINER'S TIPS

❶ By slightly changing the position of your hug, you can soothe different areas of your back. Give it a try.

❷ Beware: this stretch is so comforting you may lose track of time and just stay there!

Hip-Flexor Stretch

Hold for 20 seconds

Many people suffer from tightness in the hip flexor muscles – the muscles at the front of the thigh at hip level – which can lead to lower-back pain. Desk-bound workers can experience this, when the hip-flexors shorten and force the spine into a forward curve. This exercise really stretches the hip-flexor muscle.

Sit upright on the ball and look straight ahead. Pull your navel in towards your spine and place your hands on the tops of your thighs. Make sure you sit 'tall'.

Bring your right leg round to the back of the ball and then straighten it. Push your hips forward slightly. Your left leg should remain bent. Hold, then repeat with the other leg.

TRAINER'S TIPS
❶ Use your abdominal muscles to hold your back in a stable position and prevent your spine arching.
❷ If you feel unbalanced, rest your hands on the sides of the ball.

Toe Tilts

Hold for 30 seconds

Toe Tilts stretch deep into the muscles at the backs of the legs (the calves and the hamstrings) and are particularly useful for walkers and athletes. For desk-bound workers, long hours in a seated position can cause lower-back problems due to shortened hamstring muscles, so practise Toe Tilts regularly.

Sit upright on the ball with your knees over your feet. Rest your hands on your thighs and pull your navel in towards your spine.

Walk your feet out from the ball until your buttocks reach the edge of it. Tilt your bottom up slightly and then tilt your toes upwards. Stretch out your arms to try to touch your tilted toes, and hold. Then lower your toes, bend your knees and walk your feet back to return to the start position.

TRAINER'S TIPS

1 Keep your navel pulled in towards your spine throughout to avoid your back arching.

2 If you find it difficult to maintain your stability, position the ball against a wall.

Quad Stretch

| Hold for 30 seconds |

The fronts of the thighs are worked hard when they are exercised, so it's essential that these big, strong muscles (the quadriceps) are stretched out after being exerted. This will ensure that muscle soreness and stiffness are avoided, and the muscles will feel less tired. Quad Stretch also helps to disperse the lactic acid that forms when the legs are exercised hard.

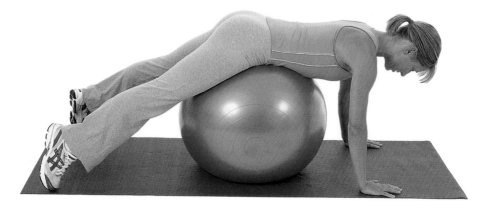

⬆ Kneel in front of the ball. Roll over the ball and 'walk out' with your hands until your hips are resting on the ball. Pull your navel in towards your spine.

⬇ Bring your right heel towards your right buttock. Reach back with your right hand and hold your right foot. You will need to adjust your body weight to balance on just your left hand. Pull on your right foot to make the stretch as intense as you want. Hold, then let go of your foot and carefully return to the start position. Repeat with the other leg.

TRAINER'S TIPS
1. Look down to the floor to maintain head and spine alignment.
2. Do not allow your back to sag.
3. This movement really challenges your balance. If you find it too demanding, use the Leg Lengthener (see page 25) as an alternative.

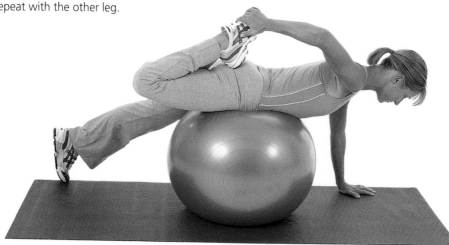

Saddle Stretch

Hold for 30 seconds

This relaxing stretch targets the adductor muscles of the inner thigh. Tightness in the inner thigh is a common problem that can lead to injury from the simplest of normal daily actions. The Saddle Stretch gets to exactly the right area, to lengthen out these naturally weaker muscles and promote greater flexibility.

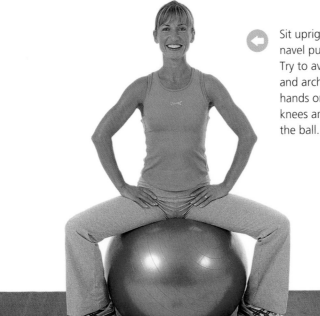

Sit upright on the ball with your navel pulled in towards your spine. Try to avoid sinking into your hips and arching your back. Place your hands on your hips and take your knees and feet out to the sides of the ball.

113

TRAINER'S TIPS
1 If you wobble, don't take your feet so far behind the ball.
2 To intensify the stretch, push your hips forward very slightly when you are in the stretched position.

Slowly slide your right foot around the side of the ball, then slide your left foot around the opposite side. Your toes must be behind the ball and in contact with the floor. Hold the stretch, then return one foot at a time to the start position.

Triceps Stretch

Hold for 10 seconds

Strong, flexible muscles at the backs of your arms are not only attractive but also help to prevent tension being stored in the chest and upper-back area. This easy-to-perform stretch improves mobility and flexibility in the shoulder area. The movement provides a real tonic for weary arms.

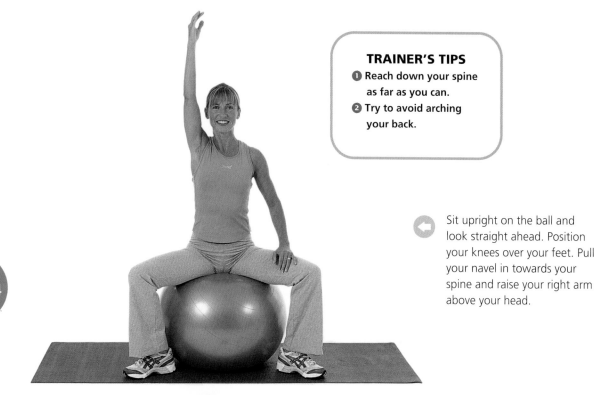

TRAINER'S TIPS
1. Reach down your spine as far as you can.
2. Try to avoid arching your back.

Sit upright on the ball and look straight ahead. Position your knees over your feet. Pull your navel in towards your spine and raise your right arm above your head.

114

Bend your right arm backwards and reach down your spine with your hand. Place your left hand on the back of your right arm. Press gently until you feel the stretch. Hold, then repeat on the other side.

Megachallenge!
To increase the intensity of the stretch gradually, grip a towel behind your back between your hands. Progressively walk your lower hand up the towel.

Seated Shoulder Smoother

**Hold for
10 seconds**

This simple stretch eases the tension and tightness often stored in the shoulders. Regular stretching provides damage limitation for vulnerable areas. This stretch will help you to unwind and de-stress at the end of a busy day.

TRAINER'S TIP
Keep your shoulders relaxed – do not hunch them!

Sit on the ball and bring your right arm across your chest with the elbow slightly bent. Place your left hand on your right upper arm and press gently to stretch. Hold. Repeat on the other side.

Kneeling Shoulder Smoother

**Hold for
10 seconds**

This kneeling shoulder stretch produces the same benefits as the seated version, but promotes a slightly deeper stretch throughout the whole shoulder area. It has the added advantage of lengthening the sides of the back.

115

Kneel with the ball in front of you, and place your hands on either side of it. Pull your navel in towards your spine.

Sit back on your heels and roll the ball away from you. Keep your arms straight and look down at the floor. Hold.

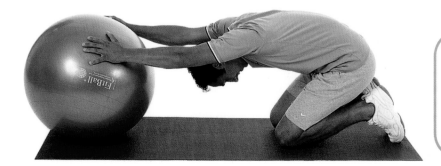

TRAINER'S TIPS
1. Do not allow your back to sag.
2. Avoid tilting your chin up.

Neck Relaxers

Hold for 1 to 2 seconds

These gentle stretches help you to relax by easing away tension from locked-up neck muscles. Stress at work or on the road can cause stiffness and neck ache that lead to headaches and weariness. Regular Neck Relaxers will promote mobility, refresh jaded concentration and make you feel rejuvenated.

Sit on the ball and pull your navel in towards your spine. Position your knees over your feet and rest your hands on the sides of the ball. Look straight ahead, with your chest open and shoulders relaxed. Tilt your right ear towards your right shoulder and hold. Return upright, then tilt to the left and hold. Repeat as often as is required.

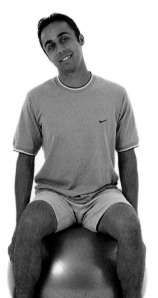

TRAINER'S TIP
Look straight ahead throughout – do not turn your head to the side when tilting.

116

From the same start position, turn your head slowly to the right and hold. Then turn to the left and hold. Repeat several times as required.

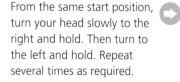

TRAINER'S TIPS
❶ Keep your head on a level plane throughout. Do not tilt your chin up or down.
❷ Turn your head to a comfortable point – never force the movement.

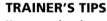

Butterfly

Hold for 20 to 30 seconds

This superb stretch achieves a wonderful extension throughout the length of the whole body. It opens and stretches the front wall of the spine, neck, arms, back and legs, inducing a sense of complete relaxation – the ultimate stretch for 'letting go'!

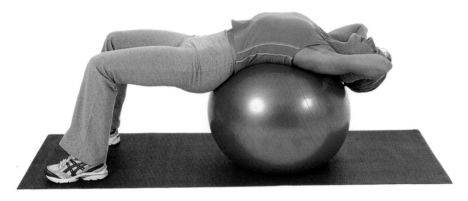

⬆ Sit on the ball with your hands placed lightly at the sides of your head. Walk your feet out until you are lying back on the ball with your neck and shoulders resting on it.

⬇ Gently arch your back over the ball, raising your arms out and over your head. Stretch your legs outwards and hold. Slowly return to the start position by walking your feet back in.

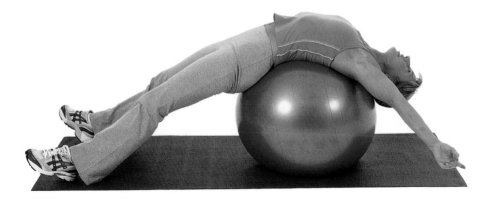

TRAINER'S TIPS
1. Avoid tensing your neck.
2. Breathe deeply to enhance your relaxation.
3. For a less intense stretch, keep your head and shoulders supported by the ball with your eyeline to the ceiling.

Scissor Stretch

Hold for 30 seconds

Lengthening the backs of the legs, the Scissor Stretch helps reduce muscle stiffness following exercise. Lower-back problems often stem from shortened hamstrings – commonly caused by too many hours spent sitting still – so it is important to keep these muscles flexible. You can adjust this stretch to suit your own flexibility and comfort.

Lie on your back with your knees slightly bent and feet hip-width apart. Hold the ball with both hands and place it on the front of your left thigh. Scissor your right leg over the top of the ball. Hold. Return to the start position and repeat on the other side.

118

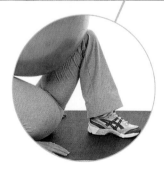

TRAINER'S TIPS
1. Allow time for your leg to relax into the stretch.
2. Breathe slowly during the stretch and relax.
3. To make the stretch less intense, straighten your lower leg a little more.

Megachallenge!
For extra intensity, bend your lower leg more by bringing your heel closer to your buttocks.

Cross-Scissor Stretch

Hold for 30 seconds

The Cross-Scissor provides a first-class stretch for the outer hips, thighs and buttocks. This gentle stretching increases flexibility, which helps to alleviate lower-back stiffness. The Cross-Scissor is a valuable stretch whether used as a cool-down after exercising or as a general relaxation technique.

Lie on your back with your knees slightly bent and feet hip-width apart. Hold the ball in both hands and place it on the front of your right thigh.

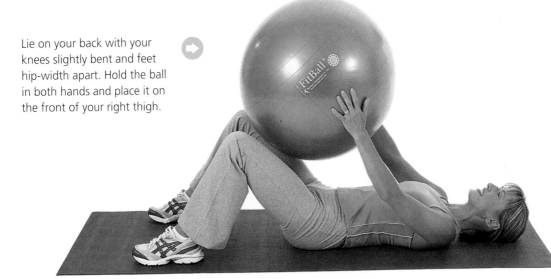

Continue to hold the ball with your hands as you scissor your left leg over the ball. Allow your left leg to roll over the top of the ball, until you feel a stretch on the outside of your left hip and thigh area. Hold. Return to the start position and repeat with the other leg.

TRAINER'S TIPS

1 Avoid forcing the stretch – ease into it slowly.
2 For increased intensity, bend the underneath leg more by bringing your heel closer to your buttocks.

119

workouts for women

Starting out

Use this total body workout programme twice a week. Perform one to two sets of each toning exercise and leave a minimum of 48 hours rest period between workouts. Before you start make sure you have read the introduction, particularly the essential advice in Getting Started, Training Guidelines and Setting Goals. This will help you to achieve the best possible results in the time you have available. Do not be put off by the long list of exercises: the warm-up exercises, for example, will only take about 5 minutes. Make notes in your fitness diary of exercises completed to keep track of your progress and help you reach your goals.

warm-up exercises

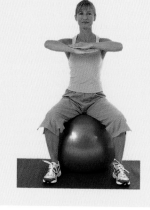

- ○ Body Balancer   p16
- ○ Shoulder Rolls   p18
- ○ Twisters   p20
- ○ Rock'n'Roll   p21
- ○ Revolver   p22
- ○ Rainbow   p23
- ○ Rear Leg Stretch   p24
- ○ Hip Lunge   p26

toning exercises

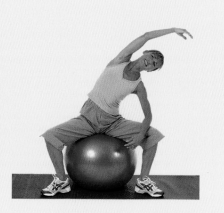

- ○ Ball Press-Up   p38
- ○ Reach for the Sky   p42
- ○ Elevator   p81
- ○ Wall Crawl   p88
- ○ Ball Drag   p82
- ○ Lean Lats   p58
- ○ Ab-Activator   p74
- ○ Overhead Triceps Press   p48
- ○ Hammer Curl   p51
- ○ Basic Ab-Fab   p66
- ○ Body Bow   p60
- ○ Basic Ab-Fab Twists   p67
- ○ Abductor Constructor   p90
- ○ Bellows   p93

cool-down stretches

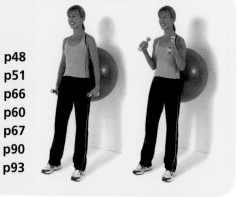
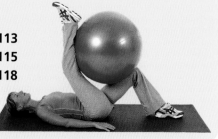

- ○ Archway   p104
- ○ Crescent Stretch   p106
- ○ Hip-Flexor Stretch   p110
- ○ Toe Tilts   p111
- ○ Saddle Stretch   p113
- ○ Shoulder Smoothers   p115
- ○ Scissor Stretch   p118

Moving on

As you become fitter, stronger and more confident, your body will need to be challenged to progress, so use this programme 3 times a week. Perform 2 to 3 sets of each toning exercise and leave a minimum of 48 hours between workouts. If you are pressed for time you may like to divide your workouts into 4 shorter sessions. For example: Monday and Friday – lower body and back exercises, and Tuesday and Thursday – upper body and stomach exercises. Add or omit exercises according to your individual needs and goals.

warm-up exercises

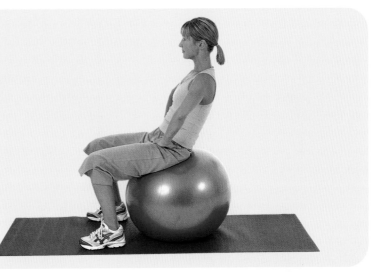

- ○ Shoulder Rolls   p18
- ○ Ball Bounce   p19
- ○ Twisters   p20
- ○ Rock'n'Roll   p21
- ○ Revolving '8'   p22
- ○ Rear Leg Stretch   p24
- ○ Upper-Back
  Stretch   p27
- ○ Leg Lengthener   p25
- ○ Look Away   p29

toning exercises

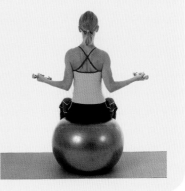

- ○ Chest Flyes   p37
- ○ Shoulder Shapers   p46
- ○ Static Wall Crawl   p89
- ○ Ball Frog   p86
- ○ Lean Lats   p58
- ○ Abs-olutely
  Fabulous   p68
- ○ Flabby-Arm
  Farewell   p47
- ○ Hammer Curl   p51
- ○ Wing Beats   p45
- ○ Reverse Curls   p71
- ○ Human Cannonball   p61
- ○ Waist Whittler   p70
- ○ Inner-Thigh Eraser   p92
- ○ Abductor Rotator   p91

cool-down stretches

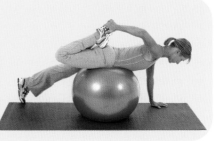

- ○ Banana Bend   p107
- ○ Toe Tilts   p111
- ○ Quad Stretch   p112
- ○ Saddle Stretch   p113
- ○ Kneeling Shoulder
  Smoother   p115
- ○ Butterfly   p117
- ○ Cross-Scissor Stretch p119

workouts for men

Starting out

Use this total body workout programme twice a week, leaving a minimum of 48 hours rest period between workouts. Before you start make sure you have read the introduction, particularly the essential advice in Getting Started, Training Guidelines and Setting Goals. This will help you to achieve the best possible results in the time you have available. Do not be put off by the long list of exercises: the warm-up exercises, for example, will take only about 5 minutes. Make notes in your fitness diary of exercises completed to keep track of your progress and help you reach your goals.

warm-up exercises

- ○ Shoulder Rolls   p18
- ○ Twisters   p20
- ○ Rock'n'Roll   p21
- ○ Ball Bounce   p19
- ○ Rainbow   p23
- ○ Rear Leg Stretch   p24
- ○ Hip Lunge   p26

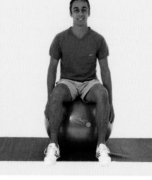

strengthening exercises

- ○ Ball Press-Up   p38
- ○ Prone Ball Row   p57
- ○ Wall Crawl   p88
- ○ Ball Drag   p82
- ○ Lean Lats   p58
- ○ Ab-Activator   p74
- ○ Drop Dips   p49
- ○ Hammer Curl   p51
- ○ Basic Ab-Fabs   p66
- ○ Body Bow   p60
- ○ Kickstart   p76
- ○ Abductor Constructor   p90
- ○ Bellows   p93

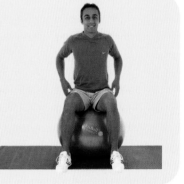

cool-down stretches

- ○ Archway   p104
- ○ Banana Bend   p107
- ○ Hip-Flexor Stretch   p110
- ○ Toe Tilts   p111
- ○ Saddle Stretch   p113
- ○ Triceps Stretch   p114
- ○ Scissor Stretch   p118

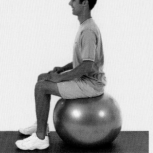
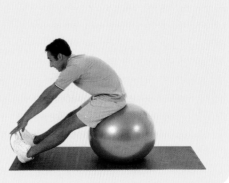

Moving on

As you become fitter, stronger and more confident, use this programme 3 times a week. Perform 2 to 3 sets of each strengthening exercise, leaving a minimum of 48 hours between each workout. If you are pressed for time you may like to divide your workouts into 4 shorter sessions. For example: Monday and Friday – lower body and back exercises, and Tuesday and Thursday upper body and stomach exericises. Add or omit exercises according to your individual needs and goals.

warm-up exercises

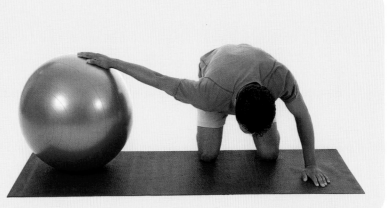

- ○ Shoulder Rolls   p18
- ○ Bouncing Jacks   p19
- ○ Twisters   p20
- ○ Rock'n'Roll   p21
- ○ Rear Leg Stretch   p24
- ○ Hip Lunge   p26
- ○ Upper-Back Stretch   p27
- ○ Chest Openers   p28

strengthening exercises

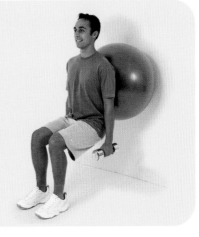

- ○ Chest Press   p40
- ○ Shoulder Glider   p59
- ○ Wall Crawl Megachallenge   p88
- ○ Single-Leg Ball Drag   p84
- ○ Wing Beats   p45
- ○ Overhead Triceps Press   p48
- ○ Biceps Curl   p50
- ○ Abs-olutely Fabulous   p68
- ○ Supaman   p54
- ○ Reverse Curls   p71
- ○ Human Cannonball   p61
- ○ Ab-Fab Twists   p69
- ○ Abductor Rotator   p91
- ○ Inner-Thigh Eraser   p92

cool-down stretches

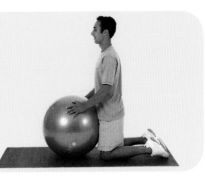

- ○ Torso Stretch   p108
- ○ Quad Stretch   p112
- ○ Saddle Stretch   p113
- ○ Triceps Stretch Megachallenge   p114
- ○ Shoulder Smoothers   p115
- ○ Neck Relaxers   p116
- ○ Cross-Scissor Stretch   p119

workout for mature people

This programme offers a range of gentle exercises designed to enhance mobility and provide essential strength and flexibility. It is suitable for mature, overweight or very unfit people. It will enable your muscles to gain strength without placing too much stress on the joints. It's always a good idea to select light weights when using dumb-bells.

Build your strength gradually, starting with twice weekly workouts. Perform 1–2 sets of each toning exercise. Leave 48 hours between workouts. When you feel stronger and more confident, add another session to your weekly programme. Make notes in your fitness diary of exercises completed to keep track of your progress and help you reach your goals.

warm-up exercises

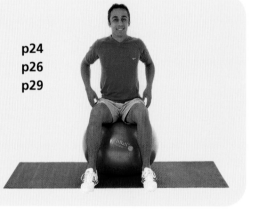

○ Body Balancer	p16	○ Rear Leg Stretch	p24
○ Shoulder Rolls	p18	○ Hip Lunge	p26
○ Twisters	p20	○ Look Away	p29
○ Rock'n'Roll	p21		
○ Revolver	p22		
○ Rainbow	p23		

toning exercises

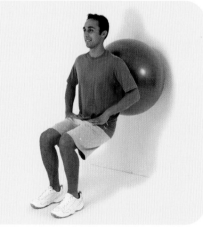

○ Arm Circles	p41	○ Hammer Curl	p51
○ Prone Ball Row	p57	○ Huggaball	p64
○ Wall Press-Up	p39	○ Basic Ab-Fabs	p66
○ Wall Crawl	p88	○ Body Bow	p60
○ Elevator	p81	○ Knee Lifts	p97
○ Reach for the Sky	p42	○ Wall Slide	p96
○ Overhead Triceps Press	p48	○ Heel Hoists	p99

cool-down stretches

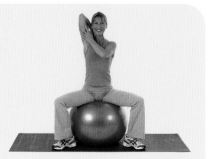
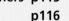

○ Archway	p104	○ Toe Tilts	p111
○ Tension Tamer	p105	○ Triceps Stretch	p114
○ Banana Bend	p107	○ Shoulder Smoothers	p115
○ Torso Stretch	p108	○ Neck Relaxers	p116
○ Lower-Spine Soother	p109		

workout for back care

Back problems are woefully neglected in many exercise programmes. A regular workout of exercises that target muscles in the back and improve strength in the deep-seated abdominal muscles will give you a strong back and central girdle. It will also improve your posture.

Use this workout twice a week to begin with and as you gain strength, add another session. You can also use this workout as a supplement to your regular programme. Perform 1–2 sets of each toning exercise, leaving 48 hours between workouts.

Always select light weights when using dumb-bells. Make notes in your fitness diary of exercises completed to keep track of your progress and help you reach your goals. If you have back problems, consult your doctor before starting this plan.

warm-up exercises

- ○ Body Balancer — p16
- ○ Ab-Engagers — p17
- ○ Ball Bounce — p19
- ○ Twisters — p20
- ○ Rock'n'Roll — p21
- ○ Revolver — p22
- ○ Rainbow — p23
- ○ Upper-Back Stretch — p27
- ○ Look Away — p29

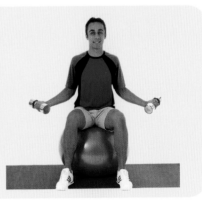

strengthening exercises

- ○ Arm Circles — p41
- ○ Shoulder Shapers — p46
- ○ Prone Ball Row — p57
- ○ Huggaball — p64
- ○ Lean Lats — p58
- ○ Ab-Activator — p74
- ○ Basic Ab-Fabs — p66
- ○ Shoulder Glider — p59
- ○ Reverse Curls — p71
- ○ Supaman — p54
- ○ Basic Ab-Fab Twists — p67
- ○ Body Bow — p60

cool-down stretches

- ○ Archway — p104
- ○ Tension Tamer — p105
- ○ Banana Bend — p107
- ○ Torso Stretch — p108
- ○ Lower-Spine Soother — p109
- ○ Hip-Flexor Stretch — p110
- ○ Kneeling Shoulder Smoother — p115
- ○ Neck Relaxers — p116
- ○ Scissor Stretch — p118

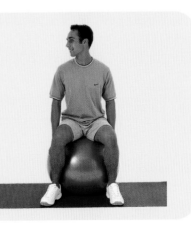

index

index and acknowledgements

Acknowledgements

I want to say a big thank you to Michael Harrison for his help and support in the writing of this book. Thanks also to my clients, whose enthusiasm for my teaching methods, particularly with the stability ball, has been an inspiration. My appreciation goes to the team at Hamlyn for their guidance and help, and to Peter Pugh-Cook for his superb photography. A special thanks goes to my family for their constant patience and support.

Executive editor Jane McIntosh
Editor Alice Tyler
Executive art editor Joanna MacGregor
Designer Ginny Zeal
Production Controller Manjit Sihra
Photography Peter Pugh-Cook
Models Jan Endacott and Karl Harrison

With special thanks to the 'Physical Company' for the kind loan of their equipment.
Physical Company
2a Desborough Industrial Park
Desborough Park Road, High Wycombe
Bucks HP12 3BG
Tel: 01494 769222
www.physicalcompany.co.uk